PSYCHOTROPIC DRUG PRESCRIBER'S SURVIVAL GUIDE

PSYCHOTROPIC DRUG PRESCRIBER'S SURVIVAL GUIDE

Ethical Mental Health Treatment
in the Age of Big Pharma

STEVEN L. DUBOVSKY, M.D.
AMELIA N. DUBOVSKY

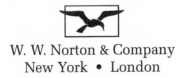

W. W. Norton & Company
New York • London

For information about permission to
reproduce selections from this book, write to
Permissions, W. W. Norton & Company, Inc.,
500 Fifth Avenue, New York, NY 10110

Production Manager: Leeann Graham
Manufacturing by Malloy Printing

Library of Congress Cataloging-in-Publication Data

Dubovsky, Steven L.
Psychotropic drug prescriber's survival guide : ethical mental health
treatment in the age of big pharma / by Steven L. Dubovsky and
Amelia N. Dubovsky—1st ed.
        p.   cm.
"A Norton professional book."
Includes bibliographical references and index.
ISBN-13: 978-0-393-70510-2
ISBN-10: 0-393-70510-2
  1. Psychotropic drugs.   2. Psychotropic drugs—testing.
3. Psychotropic drugs industry.   4. Drugs—Prescribing.
I. Dubovsky, Amelia N., 1979–.   II. Title
[DNLM: 1. Mental disorders—drug therapy.   2. Drug Therapy—
ethics.   3. Drug Industry—ethics.   4. Prescriptions, Drug—
economics.   5. Physician's Practice Patterns—ethics.
6. Advertising—ethics. WM 402 D818p 2007]

RM315.D878 2007
615'.788—dc22   2006027067

W. W. Norton & Company, Inc., 500 Fifth Avenue,
New York, N.Y. 10110
www.wwnorton.com

W. W. Norton & Company Ltd., Castle House,
75/76 Wells St., London W1T 3QT

1   3   5   7   9   0   8   6   4   2

Inspired by the courage and fortitude
of Anne Dubovsky.

CONTENTS

ACKNOWLEDGMENTS

We are grateful to Michael McGandy and Deborah Malmud for their help with this and other projects and to the faculty of the University at Buffalo Department of Psychiatry for developing innovative approaches to the interaction of industry and academia.

PSYCHOTROPIC DRUG PRESCRIBER'S SURVIVAL GUIDE

INTRODUCTION

WHY ANOTHER BOOK
ON DRUG COMPANIES?

The engaging woman was shown into my office by my secre-
tary. With a friendly smile, she informed me that she was an
MSL (medical services liaison). In response to concerns about
drug company marketing, industry had split off its marketing division consisting of the detailers or representatives who visit
every physician's office and whose job it is to market the company's products. A separate group had been created whose job it
was to meet the educational needs of the profession. As an MSL,
she was not here to sell me anything. Her mission was to provide
any information I might need about the specialty. She then pro-
ceeded to give me a colorful chart summarizing an unpublished
study of her product. Next, she handed me a couple of articles
on studies of the product but said for copyright reasons she
could not let me keep them. So she would have to summarize
the findings, which were in her view that her drug was highly effective for psychosis. Finally, she said that her product, an antipsychotic drug, was not being marketed for a particular indication
because of "a boxed—not a black box" warning, but I still might
find it useful.

As I sat there wondering why I had spent the last 30 minutes
acting as if this was actually an exchange of information even
though I had not said a word, I told her that for someone who
was not from the marketing division, she was an excellent salesperson. Proving me right, she told me how much she needed my
input about how clinicians view her product and what new uses
for it might be studied. "You're my eyes and ears," she told me,
making me feel like I was part of an important team that valued
my opinion. When she left, I did not think that her visit had af-

fected my opinion of the medication, but I had already spent more time thinking and talking about the product than I had in the previous 6 months.

At around this time, I began attending a weekly morning meeting of the clinical staff of a local hospital. At each meeting, representatives of a different drug company presented information about their product, sometimes urging the staff to discuss the good experiences they had had with the medication. A breakfast consisting of some muffins, a few slices of fruit, and a carton of orange juice supplied by the representative accompanied each presentation. After a few weeks, I asked the group why they allowed these marketing sessions to intrude into the time available for them to discuss clinical issues. The answer was that otherwise they would have to buy their own breakfast, and they were not listening anyway. I remarked rather facetiously that if they were going to sell their time for breakfast, they could at least hold out for bacon and eggs. At the next week's meeting, there it was: bacon and eggs.

When a colleague informed me that an industry representative told him over dinner (paid for by the representative) that I had said that the representative's product was the only one in its class that was effective for anxiety (something I never said), we decided to research the extent to which marketing pressures are brought to bear on our time, our attention, and ultimately our clinical judgment. We found a number of popular books, not to mention numerous articles, ranging from reasoned arguments to polemics, all recommending that marketing by the pharmaceutical industry should be severely curtailed or eliminated and that the industry as a whole should be more tightly regulated. Wondering if such draconian recommendations were any more likely to be implemented (or useful) than eliminating marketing to automobile parts dealers by manufacturers or of automobiles to the public, we did not come across anything that told us clinicians how to deal with the marketing that is part of our everyday lives and that emerges from a necessary symbiosis between our discipline and industry. This book is meant to meet such a need.

WHY ARE PEOPLE CONCERNED
ABOUT INDUSTRY INFLUENCE?

"Big pharma," the collective name for the biggest drug companies (Angell, 2005), has become an increasingly influential player in the health care field. There is one pharmaceutical sales representative, with a budget of about $100,000 each, for every 11 practicing physicians (Whiteway, 2001). Overall, drug companies spend as much as $21 billion per year promoting their products (Brennan et al., 2006; Ziegler, Lew, & Singer, 1995), and 90% of the marketing budget of big pharma is directed at physicians (Brennan et al., 2006)

Industry-sponsored research and marketing are big business, and the stakes are high. Pfizer, the world's largest pharmaceutical manufacturer and one of the largest corporations on earth, is valued at $200 billion (Moynihan & Cassels, 2005). Pfizer sales alone are around $53 billion per year, and the nine American drug companies listed in the Fortune 500 have a median profit margin of 14–19% of sales, compared with 3–5% of sales for other companies in the Fortune 500 (Angell, 2005). Americans spend more than $200 billion per year on prescription medications—a figure that does not include drugs administered to patients directly in hospitals, nursing homes, and doctors' offices (Angell, 2005).

It costs between $300 and $600 million—as much as three 747s—to bring one new drug to market (Bodenheimer, 2000). Overall, about 14% of sales go into research and development, while more than one third of pharmaceutical sales go into "marketing and administration" (Angell, 2005). The pressure to sell medications has increased as a number of "blockbuster" drugs (sales over $1 billion per year) approach the end of their patent life, without a sufficient number of potential blockbusters in the pipeline to replace them (Angell, 2005).

One way that industry has evolved to deal with the loss of the patent on a blockbuster is to develop a patentable new drug, or a new version of the existing molecule, to replace it (Angell, 2005). For example, to replace Prilosec (omeprazole), a $6 billion per year medication, the manufacturer developed a new product that consisted of the active isomer of omeprazole that they called Nexium, an apt name for a preparation that was then marketed as superior to Prilosec. A similar strategy was followed by the manufacturer of citalopram (Celexa) when its patent had only a few more years to run. Stating that it could not ethically withhold an important new development, the manufacturer licensed the S-enantomer of the drug, escitalopram (Lexapro), from another company and marketed it as superior to Celexa. The company stopped giving out Celexa samples and handed out results of a study in which depression rating scale scores were slightly lower after 1 week of treatment with Lexapro than with Celexa—a finding that was statistically significant but clinically meaningless. Thanks to the marketing efforts of the company, many clinicians had switched to the new version by the time Celexa went off patent despite lack of convincing evidence of its superiority to Celexa or any other selective serotonin reuptake inhibitor (SSRI). When Prozac (fluoxetine) lost its patent, the same drug was repackaged as Serafem, which is patented for the treatment of premenstrual dysphoric disorder at three times the price of the same dose of generic fluoxetine (Angell, 2005).

Industry-sponsored research is big business for investigators, too. As federal and foundation research dollars have become more difficult to obtain and clinical practice has become more difficult, academicians and practitioners have become more reliant on industry-sponsored activities. We will see in the next few chapters that the implications of this growing partnership are indeed profound.

Throughout the world, physicians are socialized to take part in interactions with industry representatives early in their careers. Readers who are physicians will recall who bought them their first stethoscope and doctor's bag—for most of us, it was a drug company. A survey to which 952 Finnish medical students responded found that 44% of students attended presentations by representatives at least twice a month and that students regarded industry as one of their most important sources of information about medications (Vainiomaki, Helve, & Vuorenkoski, 2004). Even though the students thought that industry promotion would affect their future prescribing habits, they were opposed to reducing promotional activities.

Although almost half of practicing physicians and one third of residents acknowledge that pharmaceutical representatives are moderately to very important in influencing their prescribing habits (Ziegler et al., 1995), many clinicians believe that they are not influenced by gifts from pharmaceutical representatives, especially if they are only small trinkets like a pen or mug. However, social science research demonstrates that the smallest gift creates a sense of obligation and that people who accept gifts with "no strings attached" still have an expectation that they should reciprocate (Brennan et al., 2006). The easiest way to repay the debt is to prescribe donor's product (Moynihan & Cassels, 2005). The more gifts that are given (e.g., food, practice aids, flattery, friendship, or empathy) and the more extensive the contact between detailer and clinician, the more likely the clinician is to identify with the commercial message (Moynihan & Cassels, 2005). Physicians' attitudes toward pharmaceutical representatives are more positive if they have received a gift from them, and physicians who request that medications be added to hospital formularies are more likely to have accepted something from a representative (Brennan et al., 2006). Accepting samples, attending industry-sponsored symposia, and even seeing representatives have been found to increase prescribing of the representative's product and requesting that the product be added to the physician's hospital formulary (Brennan et al., 2006; Somerset, Weiss, & Fahey, 2001).

The interaction of these forces with other current trends in our conceptualizations of mental disorders and their treatment has not been trivial. As managed-care protocols that only reimburse psychiatrists for writing prescriptions and not for other treatments have become the rule, the role of the psychiatrist has been narrowed to that of a prescribing machine and the relationship between the psychiatrist and the pharmaceutical industry has acquired an even more central role in the professional life of the psychiatrist (Healy, 1999). As other mental health practitioners get prescribing privileges, they may also find their roles constricting at the same time that their interactions with industry expand. No matter how strongly clinicians may feel that they are immune to economic and marketing pressures, this trend is already apparent in public settings in which nurse practitioners with prescribing authority, who are making up for a shortage of psychiatrists, are in fact doing the same thing psychiatrists do in these settings: Writing prescriptions while other clinicians provide psychological care.

And how are prescriptions for psychiatric disorders conceptualized? The early monoamine theory of depression was based on observations that reserpine caused depression and antidepressants like imipramine increased monoamine levels. However, even these early observations were complicated in that reserpine was shown in a controlled study to *be* an antidepressant, while some antidepressants (e.g., mianserin) were found to have no effects on monoamine transmission (Healy, 1999) and tianeptine, a tricyclic antidepressant used widely in France, increases monoamine (in this case, serotonin) reuptake and reduces serotonin neurotransmission (Dubovsky, 1994). The rapid ascendance of a theory that had mixed empirical support emerged from a single observed action of a few medications and "an emerging eclipse of clinical observation by laboratory based worldviews" (Healy, 1999, p. 177).

The term *antidepressant*, which appeared for the first time in the mid-1960s, was a response to reports of the antidepressant properties of the antituberculosis drug, iproniazid, and imipramine, the first synthesized antidepressant, discovered in an attempt to find a new version of chlorpromazine. Initially, the manufacturers of these medications did not see a market for the drugs because it was thought that there were no more than 50 to 100 people per million who had the kind of disorder that the new agents would treat; sales of antidepressants were in fact weak when they were first introduced (Healy, 1999). The belief that depression is common in the community only became prominent in the United States during the 1980s with the publication of landmark epidemiologic studies, which happened to be around the time that the SSRIs were developed. Although fluoxetine was the first SSRI to be introduced into the U.S. market, in 1987, zimelidine was the first medication in this class to be patented and inalpine was the first to be released (in Europe) (Healy, 1999). As treatments that were easier to use and better tolerated than the tricyclic antidepressants entered the market, more prevalence studies were conducted that showed that depression was more common than was originally thought.

The SSRIs are more consistently effective for obsessive-compulsive disorder than depression, and they are also effective for anxiety disorders and a number of other conditions. Their designation as antidepressants is primarily a function of a marketing decision. It might have been difficult to promote the SSRIs for anxiety disorders in the 1980s because public concerns about the benzodiazepines could have been transferred to the new class of medication. At the same time, estimates of the prevalence of depression increased from 100 cases per million to 50,000–100,000 cases per million (Healy, 1999), indicating a large potential market. Presentations of research demonstrating statistically dramatic effects on depression rating scale scores made the new treatments look like they were all that was necessary to treat depression. Ironically, the notion that early antidepressant treatment would reduce suicide rates and improve quality of life did not include careful monitoring of the patient by the prescriber, even though temperament and personality account for up to 50% of the variance in antidepressant response (Healy, 1999). Widespread marketing of this idea helped move psychiatry into the "brain based" era and away from a true "biopsychosocial" model, or as some have said, from the brainless psychiatry of the past to the mindless psychiatry of the present.

Industry has not only helped to set the broad conceptual framework of modern psychopharmacology, it has influenced prescribing choices. To cite just a few examples, between 1994 and 1996, prescriptions for valproate over lithium and carbamazepine in New York State increased 19-fold (Geddes & Goodwin, 2001). This increase is largely attributable to effective marketing of the product despite limited evidence at the time of effectiveness as a maintenance treatment (Geddes & Goodwin, 2001) and despite overwhelming data making lithium a more established mood stabilizer: a review of 111 class A controlled trials examined which medications had two or more placebo controlled studies (the Food and Drug Administration [FDA] criterion for approval of any indication) showing that it met one or more of the four definitions of a mood stabilizer—treating mania and depression acutely and preventing manic and depressive recurrences (Bauer & Mitchner, 2004). Only lithium met all four criteria.

The FDA prohibits marketing by industry representatives of unapproved indications for medications, and this includes just about everything in child psychiatry except for the treatment of attention deficit disorder (ADD), Tourette's syndrome, and enuresis. But there is no prohibition on the dissemination in industry-sponsored symposia or lectures of opinions of leading clinicians or the distribution of small studies and reports of open treatment of small numbers of patients. Primed by a lack of effective treatments for a growing number of serious conditions, promotion of new things to try has led to a rapid move to the use of complex and potentially dangerous drug combinations for childhood mood and behavioral disorders in the absence of any scientific support at all for most applications (March, Silva, Compton, Califf, & Krishnan, 2005) and without adequate support for many adult applications. This outcome requires clinicians to be more vigilant for new data about experimental uses of medications.

Recently, a new player has entered the psychiatric marketplace: the manufacturer of the medical device. The vagus nerve stimulator (VNS) was recently approved for the treatment of refractory depression. Empirical support for this use of VNS, which costs around $20,000 to implant and includes a charge of over $100 each time the stimulus is adjusted, comes from a study showing that 29% of patients with chronic or recurrent depression who had failed to respond to four treatment trials responded (40–50% improvement in Hamilton Depression Rating Scale [HDRS or HAM-D] scores) to a VNS after 9 to 12 months of treatment, although a 3-month double-blind study showed no effect and with chronic treatment 30 of 205 patients got worse and 7 attempted suicide (3 for the first time) (Rush, 2005). Not surprisingly, seminars and articles supported by the manufacturer began to proliferate in anticipation of approval of the device and opportunities for exposure to information about

VNS now abound. While we will not discuss this and other devices with potential applications in psychiatry, the principles of dealing with marketing them are the same as for pharmaceutical agents.

IS THE PHARMACEUTICAL
INDUSTRY THE EVIL EMPIRE?

Marketing is inevitable in every field of endeavor, and medicine is no exception. But is it as pernicious as it is pervasive? A recent proposal for reform of the relationship between academic medical centers and industry provided a long list of activities that were felt to have the potential to influence physician behavior in a way that could supersede the needs of the patient (Brennan et al., 2006). These authors suggested prohibiting any gifts, even of small items, as well as all meals, payment for attendance at lectures and conferences, direct industry support of any continuing medical education (CME), payment for time and travel while at meetings, participation in speakers bureaus, putting one's name on any ghostwritten article, and accepting drug samples. Paid consultation was acceptable if a specific work product of the consultation was specified, but research grants would only be permitted if they were unrestricted, thereby prohibiting participation of academic faculty in development of new medications for FDA approval and other commercial purposes.

While this global restriction of industry–academic interactions might reduce some of the more blatant influences discussed later of marketing on thought leaders in psychiatry and therefore on the field, the wisdom of prohibiting all marketing is open to discussion. In a free society, is it better to prohibit anything that might influence prescribing, or to teach clinicians how to deal with such pressures? Should anything that can influence decision makers be eliminated in all fields? What about marketing of ideas having nothing to do with industry by experts that are supported more by the experts' opinion than hard data or that should be balanced by contradictory theories? Should marketing of and providing samples of automobile parts to repair shops and dealerships be prohibited because it could influence the recipient's choice of product toward more expensive or even inferior parts? Should all advertising be prohibited that could influence decision makers whose decisions affect others such as airline executives or stockbrokers?

Currently, more than half of all clinical research is supported by drug companies (Healy & Thase, 2003), and even if the basic work is funded by the federal government and performed in universities, virtually all new compounds are developed and tested clinically by industry. It is impossible to estimate how many patients would suffer without the investment of industry in developing and distributing new treatments (Brennan et al., 2006). While the interpretation of industry-sponsored research can be open to considerable question, it at least produces data, which independent sources can then address (Smith, 1998).

A number of influential experts have advocated attempts to separate marketing from other aspects of industry effort on the grounds that big pharma has a profound impact on public welfare. Such opinions minimize the reality that many things that impact on public health, from academic activities to government initiatives to the ideas of experts, involve producing a product that in one way or another is marketed to decision makers. Theories that are marketed to grant review committees, ideas that are marketed to colleagues and editors of prestigious journals, and opinions that are marketed to the public in order to promote a political agenda all have the same potential as the marketing of pharmaceutical industry products to influence prescribing habits, public health, and even our basic safety. Whether the reward be sales, prestige, grant funding, or votes, all marketing has a potential payoff. Knowing what that payoff is helps the consumer of information to interpret the marketing without eliminating the dissemination of ideas and opinions.

There is very little in a free society that is not subject to overstatement, overinterpretation, or even falsification. Protecting the public from such exaggerations by attempting to legislate away industry marketing may not even be effective if professionals and their patients are still inclined to accept ideas uncritically because they are published in an important journal or promulgated by a nationally recognized expert. The primary theme of this book is that marketing is ubiquitous, and the only thing that pretending to separate it from other scientific initiatives will accomplish is to relieve clinicians of the obligation to think critically about all of the information to which they are exposed by leading them to believe that they can defer scientific inquiry to the experts. We may be more effective at protecting our patients from overenthusiastic marketing by learning how to identify and interpret it than by delegating to others the responsibility of deciding what to do about the marketing to which we will continue to be exposed so long as we are in a marketplace economy.

WHAT TO EXPECT FROM
THIS BOOK

Clinicians depend on continually updated information from multiple sources in order to prescribe responsibly. This book will provide a framework for identifying how new findings are developed and marketed. After reviewing how industry research works and how it influences clinical practice, we will examine the wide role played by industry marketing in all domains of mental health practice. We will learn basic principles of research and we will have the opportunity to apply those principles to some influential studies that influence our standard of care. After a brief tutorial on basic marketing, we will learn how to deal with the marketing to which we are exposed every day in our offices, clinics, and hospitals. By the end of the book, you will be able to use scientific principles to interpret both good and bad effects of the treatments you use and to apply scientific principles to the mass of information with which we are continually deluged.

Fundamentals

I

The Growing Role of Industry in Psychiatry

1

Industry has become inextricably entwined in psychiatric research, education, and practice. Let's examine how this has occurred in each of these domains.

RESEARCH

Conducting clinical studies of new and established products that are still on patent is a core industry activity that is discussed in detail in Chapter 3. Two events have greatly increased the importance of this activity to the profession. First, as the potential market for new products has expanded, so has the number of studies designed to gain approval for new drugs or to support new uses of existing products that have reached the limit of market penetration for the indication for which they were initially approved. To conduct more research, pharmaceutical manufacturers have had to find more investigators who are able to recruit sufficient numbers of patients to complete clinical trials.

The second important change has been a decrease in the availability of federal funds for clinical investigation. Funding from the national institutes has not kept up with the growing number of projects that are indicated by advances in science, and it is expected to decrease at a time when more academic institutions are competing for federal funding, in order to advance knowledge as well as their standing in the profession. With a decreasing pool of federal funds, industry-sponsored trials have become an attractive source of flexible income that can be used to support the overall research infrastructure and the salaries of investigators and their personnel. Competition has therefore increased for these funds as well.

Industry spending on research grants to investigators increased from $3.2 billion in 1994 to $22 billion in 2004 (i.e., by $19 billion) (Warner & Roberts, 2004), but the percentage of research going to academic medical centers decreased over the same time from 63% to 26% (Steinbrook, 2005a). The reason for this dramatic change is that industry has recruited more researchers of its own to design and conduct research, and more community physicians have gotten into the business of research (Bodenheimer, 2000). In contrast, National Institutes of Health (NIH) research funding increased from $4.5 billion to $13.9 billion (i.e., by $9 billion) between 1985 and 1999 (Warner & Roberts, 2004). The National Science Foundation spends $586 million a year on biomedical research, the Howard Hughes Medical Institute spends $573 million, and the American Cancer Society spends $131 million (Cech, 2005). Industry funding accounts for 57% of U.S. biomedical research, NIH for 28%, and state and local governments support just 5% of clinical investigations (Moses, Dorsey, Matheson, & Thier, 2005). In psychiatry, industry funding of research in 2000 was $4.1 billion compared with $850 million from the National Institute of Mental Health (NIMH). The FDA itself is becoming dependent on industry support. Through charges to sponsors for reviews of products submitted for approval, more than half of the FDA's review work is funded directly by the industry it reviews (Abramson, 2004).

Initially, most industry research collaborations were with universities, but as changes in third-party payment created decreased reimbursement and increased unpaid paperwork, private groups have emerged to compete for industry-sponsored clinical trials. Managed care has not yet come to industry-sponsored trials, which remain more lucrative than clinical work. At the same time, industry has become frustrated with academic investigators because their contracting and research approval processes are slow and complex and their more diverse activities make it take longer to complete a study. This is hardly a trivial matter: each additional day spent obtaining FDA approval of a drug costs $1.3 million (Bodenheimer, 2000)! This makes private groups whose only activity has become to conduct clinical trials more appealing unless the academic investigator has unique expertise or unique populations of patients to which no one else has access.

CONTROL OF RESEARCH DATA

The contracting process in academic centers may be difficult and time-consuming to negotiate, but the core dedication of academia to rapid and open sharing of data can be an even more important impediment to research collaborations with industry. Traditionally, data from industry-sponsored trials have been considered proprietary: the company that funded the study owns the result. Ownership of data has been easy to enforce in multicenter double-blind studies because investigators at any site do not know which treatment their subjects had, and only the sponsor has all the data. Investigators have theoretically been able to see results of the entire study, but it is usually difficult to gain access to all the data and in some instances sponsors have insisted on the power to veto or at least defer publication of results they do not like. When an industry-sponsored study is published, it is frequently written by a professional team of writers who work for the company or a lead investigator who has moved from academics to the research department of the sponsor. The conflict between the need of the sponsor to control data related to development of its product and the academician's need to publish data in the most complete form possible can make it onerous for industry to contract with academic centers.

The truth is that most of the time this conflict is not very intense. Most academic investigators who are involved in industry-sponsored research, especially studies designed to get FDA approval, realize that they are really engaging in product development, the main advantage of which for them is to generate flexible funds for other research. As a result, they are more likely to accept without comment the preparation of reports for publication by the manufacturer or its agent, and they are not as likely to be concerned if negative results are not published (Bodenheimer, 2000). Sometimes, however, disputes about publication can become rancorous. For example, when a Canadian researcher found that a drug used to treat thalassemia major could aggravate hepatic fibrosis, the manufacturer threatened legal action if the finding was published because a contract was in place forbidding disclosure of results for 3 years without the company's permission (Bodenheimer, 2000). Similarly, when a manufacturer-sponsored study found that a brand-name preparation of thyroxine was no more effective than generics, the company enforced the stipulation in the research contract that no information could be released without the company's permission (Bodenheimer, 2000). In both of these cases, the results were eventually published, but it took a considerable amount of time and involved years of legal wrangling.

In informal interviews with faculty involved with industry-sponsored research, Bodenheimer (2000) learned that all of them had experienced having research reports written or altered by the funding company. In one case, the company held up publication for 6 months while it requested revisions that cast the company's product in a more favorable light, and in the meantime it published a competing article that supported the product.

One of the first high-profile cases of limited access to data to involve psychiatry occurred when researchers who conducted industry-sponsored studies of antidepressants in children and adolescents were denied access to unpublished data from their own studies showing a relationship between these medications and increased suicidality (Steinbrook, 2005a). When, as described on page 42, an FDA employee took it upon himself to reanalyze all unpublished data on pediatric antidepressant trials, he concluded that patients taking antidepressants were about twice as likely to develop new or increased suicidal thoughts or attempt suicide than patients taking placebo. Had the data been reported initially, the risk could have been put in proper perspective and researchers could have pointed out that the overall risk was still small, that it was only manifested soon after starting the antidepressant, that no patient actually committed suicide in these trials, and that there is excellent evidence that antidepressants decrease suicide risk in younger patients. Withholding the information from public scrutiny, however, caused such an outcry that warnings were added to antidepressant labeling that have made many pediatricians and some psychiatrists reluctant to prescribe an antidepressant for patients for whom the medication might be very useful.

In 2001, the International Committee of Medical Journal Editors began to require that the primary author accept responsibility for the conduct of reported studies, have access to the data, and control the decision to publish. However, it was later demonstrated that academic institutions routinely engaged in industry-sponsored research that did not adhere to these guidelines (Steinbrook, 2005a). In 2005, the director of the Cleveland Clinic Cardiovascular Coordinating Center said that "commercial sponsors still exclusively control the database for most clinical trials" (Steinbrook, 2005a, p. 2161).

The University of Toronto instituted a policy in 2001 in which clinical research contracts cannot contain the proviso that sponsors can suppress or censor results; investigators are also supposed to be permitted to disclose safety issues immediately (Steinbrook, 2005a). This policy arose from the case of a Toronto hematologist who had a confidentiality agreement with the manufacturer of an iron chelator who was sued by the company when she tried to publish findings about lack of safety of the medication (Steinbrook, 2005a). However, the Pharmaceutical Research and Manufacturers of America's (PhRMA) guidelines stated that "sponsors have discretion to determine who will have access to the database . . . [and] will make a summary of the study results available to the investigators. In addition, any investigators who participated in the conduct of a multi-site clinical trial will be able to review relevant statistical tables, figures and reports for the entire study at the sponsor's facilities, or other mutually agreeable location" but not at their own site (Steinbrook, 2005a, p. 2162). Despite such policies, most contracting by academic medical centers for industry-sponsored research focuses on financial aspects of the contract and have no proviso for access by investigators to the body of data produced by the study (Drazen, 2002).

THE POTENTIAL FOR CONFLICTS OF INTEREST

This discussion makes it seem as if the only challenge to clinical investigators is for them to gain access to information they helped to produce in order to maintain their obligation to report research findings objectively. However, the interaction between researchers and industry is more complicated. Good researchers are successful because they design and conduct good studies, and this makes them attractive to industry, just as it does to other funding sources. For their part, many well-known investigators look to industry for flexible sources of funding for their research and for ways of augmenting their income and public exposure beyond what the traditional academic role is able to provide.

To illustrate the extent of faculty–industry interactions, a stratified random sample between 1994 and 1995 of 2,167 faculty involved in research at the 50 universities that received the most NIH research funding in 1993 was selected for a mail survey. Faculty were selected from a medicine or medicine subspecialty group, one other clinical department, and two basic science departments at each institution (Campbell, Louis, & Blumenthal, 1998), but the results are equally applicable to psychiatry faculty. Respondents were asked about gifts (independent of grants and contracts) from industry that included equipment, biomaterials, discretionary funds, trips, support for students, and other support, and about what they thought the company expected in return. Of the sample, 43% had received a gift, and the majority of these had received more than one type of gift. Clinical researchers were more likely to receive gifts than basic science faculty, and faculty who had research grants and contracts were more likely to receive gifts than faculty without grants. The more productive the researchers, the more likely they were to have received gifts. Two thirds of all faculty rated the gifts as "important," "very important," or "essential" to their research. One report even noted that 54% of consultants to FDA advisory committees had a "direct financial interest in the drug or topic they are asked to evaluate" (Abramson, 2004, p. 90).

While industry primarily develops and markets new medications, basic science discoveries that lead eventually to new pharmacologic concepts are funded by the NIH. All such discoveries were in the public domain until the Bayh-Dole Act was passed in the 1980s, which permitted universities and small business to patent discoveries that emerged from NIH-sponsored research and to then license the patents exclusively to drug companies (Angell, 2005). The act created a new kind of partnership in which paying a royalty to the university allowed industry to license a product developed with publicly funded research for a relatively modest royalty compared to the profit from marketing the product. At the same time, a growing number of investigators and universities acquired equity in new biotechnology enterprises and greater financial interest in new drug development by industry.

An example of the new industry- and taxpayer-sponsored enterprise is provided by Angell (2005). Paclitaxel (Taxol), the best-selling cancer chemotherapy drug ever, was derived from the bark of the Pacific yew tree. The National Cancer Institute (NCI) funded $183 million in research to develop paclitaxel, and 30 years after it was discovered, NCI and Bristol-Myers Squibb (BMS) signed a cooperative agreement in which the company supplied paclitaxel, which it obtained from a chemical company, to NCI for further research. After Taxol was approved by the FDA for treating refractory ovarian cancer, BMS was given a 5-year exclusive patent for the drug. When a method of synthesizing paclitaxel (instead of obtaining it from the yew tree) was developed with NIH funding at Florida State University, the university licensed the method for tens of millions of dollars in royalties to BMS, which made $1 billion to $2 billion per year from the preparation. The lesson of the profit to both members of the university–BMS partnership is obvious to other academic centers wanting to replace funding lost as a result of declining direct government support for independent research.

When we read journals these days, we often see a blurb in small print at the end of an article about the relationships of the authors with industry, so that readers can decide whether these relationships influence the content. However, journals do not always insist on such disclosures. For example, only 2 of 70 articles (mostly reviews and letters) about calcium channel antagonists disclosed the authors' potential conflicts of interest, but when contacted directly two thirds of the authors had a financial relationship with industry, and 96% of authors who supported the safety of these drugs, but only 37% of those who did not, had industry relationships (Smith, 1998). This may have been because experts who had financial relationships with manufacturers of these drugs had more experience with them, but the issue at least should be open to discussion.

A quick perusal of any issue of a major psychiatry journal will reveal either that most large studies are directly supported by industry, or that one or more authors report consulting relationships with industry or industry support of other research. In addition, the names of most of the more prominent authors will be readily recognizable because they have participated in industry-sponsored symposia or they have written articles in journal supplements supported by industry grants. These kinds of potential conflicts of interest are rarely reported. According to the *British Medical Journal (BMJ)*, authors do not always report all potential conflicts of interest because they think that these are trivial, that they will be perceived as bad, or because they think that writing or speaking for industry will not influence their findings and recommendations (Smith, 1998).

Despite increased concerns about reporting potential conflicts of interest, situations still exist in which such conflicts are deliberately concealed. In a front-page article in its April 24, 2006 issue, the *Wall Street Journal* reported (pp. A1, A12) on an article by a Harvard Medical School cardiologist in the trade publication *Physician's Weekly Journal* contending that as many as 30% of the 25 million Americans who take aspirin to reduce the risk of a heart attack develop "aspirin resistance" and need proprietary antiplatelet drugs instead. The *Physician's Weekly* article did not mention that the cardiologist had research funding from a company that makes a test to measure aspirin resistance, or that he was a consultant and paid speaker for the manufacturer of a new brand-name antiplatelet drug that would be used in cases of aspirin resistance and that he had research funding from that company as well. The managing editor of *Physician's Weekly* said that the publication never discloses potential conflicts of interest but uses the information to find companies that might want to advertise near the physician's commentary. Interestingly, the *Wall Street Journal* article pointed out that some physicians who contend that there is no such thing as aspirin resistance have financial ties to an aspirin manufacturer. Even more startling was the comment of a hematologist who has consulted to manufacturers of both aspirin and proprietary aspirin alternatives: "I try to be honest with myself, but I can't pretend I will always be as honest as possible" (p. A12). In contrast, the Harvard cardiologist argued that most researchers who do not have conflicts of interest "are not truly expert" (p. A12). The hematologist, who would be an expert by this criterion, said that a study he had done indicating that a certain urine test demonstrated that aspirin resistance could triple the risk of cardiovascular death later said that the test used "the wrong marker" (p. A12).

Regardless of what investigators believe, industry contributions to research and other professional activities of leaders in psychiatry create powerful incentives to keep the relationship going. Will the company provide more support to researchers who repeatedly point out the weaknesses of its research or who underscore the exaggerations in the marketing of its product? Will invitations to lead important symposia continue when the investigator might say at the symposia that the evidence in favor of first-line use of the sponsor's product is weak? Our academic leaders are among the most intelligent and accomplished in the world, but are they immune to human motivations?

CONSULTATION TO THE MARKET

There are increasing opportunities for physicians, not only to work with drug companies and manufacturers of medical devices, but to advise Wall Street whether to invest in their products. This is a big portion of the market: about one third of hedge fund investments and the same proportion of venture capital investments are in health care–related companies, primarily pharmaceutical, biotechnology, and medical device manufacturers (Topol & Blumenthal, 2005).

The billions of dollars involved in these investments have spawned an entire consulting industry. For example, a New York company advertises a worldwide network of more than 100,000 experts, including 60,000 physicians and 12,000 other health care professionals, who are available as consultants to investors (Steinbrook, 2005b; Topol & Blumenthal, 2005). In the United States, the number of physicians involved in these kinds of consulting relationships increased from 1,000 in 1996 to 75,000 in 2005, a 75-fold increase in just 8 years (Topol & Blumenthal, 2005). Almost 10% of American doctors have formal consulting arrangements with the investment industry, at rates from $200 to more than $1000 per hour (Anonymous, 2005). The most important focus of these consultations has been the status of ongoing clinical trials (Topol & Blumenthal, 2005). For example, in 2002 the *Wall Street Journal* reported that an investment firm learned from a physician consultant that a case of Guillain-Barré syndrome had occurred in a clinical trial of an antiobesity drug, resulting in a drastic drop in the value of the company's stock (Anand & Smith, 2002).

In August 2005, the *Seattle Times* reported having found 26 cases in which physicians leaked confidential information about ongoing drug research to Wall Street firms (Steinbrook, 2005b). Such information was then used to advise clients whether to buy stock in the company doing the research, often before results of a study are released. This kind of disclosure, which often violates the confidentiality agreement most investigators sign before undertaking an industry-sponsored clinical trial, makes the investigator invaluable to the investment firm and creates an interesting opportunity for conflicts of interest in two directions at the same time.

While experts increasingly disclose relationships to pharmaceutical companies, disclosure of relationships between experts and investment firms is rare (Topol & Blumenthal, 2005). Even when physicians do not reveal proprietary information to investment firms, these firms may advertise relationships with prominent advisers in a way that creates the impression that the firm has an inside track to important information that will maximize its investments (Topol & Blumenthal, 2005). Whether relationships with investment firms are disclosed by psychiatrists or by the firms, it is difficult to know how to manage the conflicts of interest inherent in the complexity of the relationships.

INDUSTRY AND PSYCHIATRIC EDUCATION

Advice published in the magazine *Pharmaceutical Marketing* proposed that medical education is "a potent weapon to be used by the marketer in supporting promotional activities" (Somerset et al., 2001, p. 1483). In the psychiatric setting, industry-sponsored teaching begins in medical school, intensifies during residency, and reaches its maturity in CME. It is now difficult to find practitioners who do not receive the bulk of their postgraduate exposure to new data either directly from industry representatives or in industry-sponsored programs and publications.

In the United States, 85% of residency education programs allow industry representatives to provide food for conferences and 46% permit them to give presentations; residents interact with an average of four to six representatives per month (Ziegler et al., 1995). Indeed, many programs have traditionally encouraged industry involvement with their residents as a means of providing free food, textbooks, and travel for cash-strapped trainees. In addition to reinforcing the teaching partnership of industry and medicine, sponsored activities in an educational program that provide these kinds of benefits reinforce the notion that physicians should depend on industry to buy essential items or services that previous generations bought for themselves. The concern of course is that such largesse will create a sense of dependency on industry that will generalize to a need for new information.

A study at a university-based internal medicine residency education program used an interesting method to examine the accuracy of information presented by industry representatives prior to faculty presentations at teaching conferences at which the representatives presumably provided food or other items (Ziegler et al., 1995). A pharmacist attended 15 consecutive conferences, 13 of which contained presentations by representatives prior to the faculty lecture. The average audience included 33 residents, as well as medical students rotating through the service. The faculty lectures were unrelated to the pharmaceutical representatives' presentations. The pharmacist recorded the representatives' comments, which lasted from 30 seconds to 12 minutes (average 2.4 minutes) and analyzed them for accuracy. An inaccurate statement was defined as contradicting prescribing information in the PDR, a clinical pharmacologist thought the statement was inaccurate, and there was no support for the statement in textbooks, Medline, and drug company brochures.

Of 106 representative statements that were examined, 11% were inaccurate, all in a way that favored the sponsored drug. Of the accurate statements about promoted drugs, 49% were favorable to the promoted drug, 31% were neutral, and 19% were unfavorable. Therefore, inaccurate statements were significantly more likely to cast the promoted drug in a favorable light than were accurate statements ($p = 0.005$). Overall, 56% of representatives' statements about their own drugs were favorable, but none of their statements about competing drugs were favorable. An example of an inaccurate statement about a promoted drug was "We are the only SSRI that has long-term data," when one of its competitors had longer-term data and had been on the market for 5 years versus just 3 months for the promoted drug. An even more blatant example: "Your *Medical Letter* this month has a favorable review of drug E. This is with regard to rapid hemodynamic effect of drug E after a single dose increasing cardiac index." However, a copy of the issue to which the representative referred, which was available at the talk, said that a different drug was preferred and did not mention a rapid hemodynamic effect or the cardiac index. All residents thought that the lunch with the promotion made them more likely to attend future conferences and only 26% thought that a false statement had ever been made. The vast majority of residents (85%) thought that pharmaceutical representatives provide useful information, 52% said that they sought information about drugs from industry representatives, and 37% said the information influenced their prescribing. Not one inaccurate statement by a representative was questioned by any of the residents. Almost half (44%) of the residents thought that the representatives provided more reliable information than printed advertisements, although the latter are more tightly regulated by the FDA.

CONTINUING MEDICAL EDUCATION

In 2001, industry sponsored more than 60% of CME programs, a figure that has increased since then (Angell, 2005). CME has grown exponentially with the explosion of new knowledge that is emerging, and in response to requirements by hospitals, professional societies, and some licensing boards that practitioners attend a certain number of hours of CME programs every year.

In response to the growing CME market, a proliferation of private medical education companies has been accredited by the Accreditation Council for Continuing Medical Education (AC-CME), thanks to recommendations of a task force consisting of representatives of educational institutions, professional organizations, industry, and CME companies themselves (Angell, 2005). As Angell noted, these companies fund CME activities through "unrestricted educational grants" from industry, ostensibly to ensure that the manufacturer does not exert direct influence over the content of the program. However, the program is organized around the condition treated by the sponsor's product, and a program that cast the product in an unfavorable light would not be likely to be followed by more unrestricted grants by that company. One CME company apparently told potential sponsors that "medical education is a powerful tool that can deliver your message to key audiences, and get those audiences to take action that benefits your product" (2005, p. 139).

Professional societies such as the American Psychiatric Association (APA) are the primary providers of CME for many psychiatrists. The highlight of the year's educational activities for psychiatrists is the annual APA meeting, which is heavily supported by industry. Industry-sponsored symposia, which are among the most popular presentations at the APA meeting because of the effort that goes into preparing the lectures, are a cornerstone of the meeting. Angell (2005) quotes a newspaper article pointing out that in addition to $60,000 in direct payments to the APA for the privilege of putting on each of 55 or so industry-sponsored symposia, another $400,000 was spent on the symposia themselves.

It is impressive to get to an industry-sponsored breakfast symposium at the APA meeting at 6:00 a.m. and see a line of attendees waiting to get in so they get a good seat. They know that they will hear the best speakers in the field and that they will see professionally prepared slides and handouts that present complex data in a straightforward manner. Is it altruism that leads the sponsor to put so much time and effort into these presentations, or is there enough evidence that the program will promote loyalty to the company and the product to justify the expense to its stockholders? Would any successful business spend large amounts of money on anything without evidence that the activity promoted its sales? The recognition that a good program creates more goodwill for the company and ultimately more business would result in greater dedication to completely unbiased presentation of data in other venues.

The APA is as interested in having industry-sponsored symposia at its meetings as the manufacturers are in presenting them. An obvious motivation is the preference of the members for these events. However, there is another benefit that is also important to the organization and its members. The money paid by industry for its symposia and exhibits makes the annual meeting profitable, which not only keeps the registration fee down but helps the APA to hold the line on its dues. Without this support, both dues and fees for attending the annual meeting would rise substantially.

This is not just a national phenomenon. Many APA district branches and other local professional organizations rely on industry sponsorship for many of their routine activities. Many district branch monthly meetings include talks by someone from an industry speaker's bureau. The talks may be of high or low quality, but they always focus on the company's product, or at least on the condition for which the product is prescribed. Such talks give members a handy opportunity to amass CME credits, but they have another, more essential benefit. Because everyone works during the day, the district branch usually meets in the evening, often for dinner. Thanks to the sponsor, the dinner is free. For some members, years of sponsorship of local meetings have made it inconceivable that they should have to pay for the dinners themselves. At one time, goodwill and loyalty to the company were sufficient rewards for companies to sponsor local APA meetings, but new guidelines emerging from concerns about physicians appearing to be in bed with drug companies have made it necessary for the meetings to have an educational component if the companies are to pay for the meetings. So now each meeting includes a speaker. The only problem is that industry-sponsored speakers must follow new guidelines described in the next few paragraphs that makes the dinners into promotional events.

Participating in industry-sponsored education can be an effective marketing tool for speakers as well as manufacturers. The APA now requires that one speaker at an industry-sponsored symposium be a junior faculty member, and presenting at one of these events provides an opportunity for national exposure. At the same time, established senior investigators become even better known presenting at nationally prominent events such as the APA meeting. This kind of marketing of oneself may be a more enduring incentive than an honorarium for giving an exciting talk—and for being invited back.

A related cornerstone of CME these days is the industry-sponsored dinner. At one time, local practitioners would ask a drug company to sponsor a dinner speaker who was free to prepare slides or obtain them from the manufacturer and to discuss whatever seemed reasonable. Recently, to avoid the appearance of presenting data about a product inappropriately, new PhRMA guidelines were developed that require that the presentation contain only FDA-approved information, which is essentially the information in the package insert and is the same information that industry representatives are allowed to present. The practical outcome of these guidelines is that the speaker's lecture is essentially the presentation that might be made by a sophisticated industry representative. Slides and handouts are prepared by the company, with input from experts on the topic who are well known to the company and from industry employees who check that nothing is inconsistent with FDA requirements. The speaker is free to answer questions with additional comments, but the formal presentation is sculpted by the sponsor. The manifest objective is to protect clinicians and their patients, but the result is that the most independent speaker must conform to a framework prepared by the manufacturer in order to give a dinner talk.

This kind of structure, which amounts to direct marketing, is not even necessary to achieve that goal. Years ago, the manufacturer of an antidepressant asked me to give a series of lectures of my own design on the treatment of depression in medical practice to groups of primary-care physicians. As I thought that the company's product was more appropriately used by specialists than by nonpsychiatrists, I either did not mention it or said that it was not a first-line treatment in general medical practice. Yet I kept getting asked back to give more talks. When I asked why they wanted me to speak, the industry spokesperson who arranged the talks said that for 30 days after a lecture that the participants liked, prescriptions in the region increased for all of the company's products, including its antibiotics, prescription allergy medications, and other preparations. This is apparently an established principle: Angell (2005) notes that prescriptions for Neurontin (gabapentin) by speakers who got an honorarium from the manufacturer to present at a dinner meeting increased by 70% after the meeting, undoubtedly helping Neurontin bring in $2.7 billion for the manufacturer in 2003.

NONMEDICAL PROVIDERS

Psychiatry remains a shortage specialty in many regions of the United States, and the shortage of child psychiatrists is even more acute. In some states, nurse practitioners with advanced training who have acquired prescribing authority can help to fill the gap. A collaborative agreement with a physician is usually necessary, but the nurse practitioner can essentially function as an independent prescriber. A group of psychologists has recently been pressing for prescribing privileges, and two states have granted such privileges for psychologists who take courses in psychopharmacology on the grounds that there are not enough psychiatrists to prescribe medications for psychiatric patients. Both groups represent important potential markets for industry. Initially, they have been included with psychiatrists and other physicians in industry-sponsored presentations, but as prescribing psychiatric medications becomes a more essential component of each group's professional identity, they may achieve a critical mass that deserves marketing of its own.

It will be interesting to see how not having been exposed to industry marketing during training will affect the responsiveness of nonmedical prescribers to industry marketing. Will they be even more appreciative and less critical of industry largesse, or will they be more skeptical of industry-sponsored education they have not been exposed to previously? In either case, the same principles of evaluating marketing and research data will apply.

It is not necessary to prescribe oneself in order to be a useful target of industry marketing. Many nonmedical providers advise patients about their medications, and in many organizations nurses provide formal education about medications to patients. With the dissemination of information about psychiatric treatments, it is not at all uncommon these days for therapists to advise patients to add a medication to their treatment, and often to suggest which medication to try. No wonder, then, that industry representatives bring lunches to hospitals, mental health centers, and office staff members, along with invitations to participate in educational activities.

EVIDENCE-BASED PRACTICE

One of the most influential movements in clinical medicine has been "evidence-based medicine," which presumably is the cornerstone of the clinical practice guidelines and insurance reviews that are discussed in Chapter 7. The concept of evidence-based medicine was meant to replace the traditional model of basing clinical decisions solely on one's own clinical experience, presumed pathophysiology, or the opinion of an expert with a good reputation (Group, 1992). Evidence-based medicine holds that clinical experience and intuition are essential, especially in the absence of controlled data, but they can be misleading. Similarly, rationales for diagnosis and treatment based solely on basic pathophysiology may be incorrect. The evidence-based medicine paradigm reduces the authority of experts and emphasizes that physicians should gain the skills necessary to make independent assessments of evidence and critically evaluate the opinions of experts (Group, 1992). However, a keystone of this paradigm is the assumption that the evidence itself is valid, and we will see in the next few chapters that 10 years after the widespread dissemination of the concept in psychiatry, this assumption is not yet entirely reliable.

Evidence-based guidelines are assembled by expert consensus panels who are supposed to be independent of opinion and marketing. However, an investigation of panels by the journal *Nature* that write clinical guidelines found that 35% of authors declared financial links to drug companies that make products included in the guidelines; about 70% of panels had at least one member with a conflict of interest (Reichardt, 2005). In one panel, every member had received payment from the company that manufactured the drug that the panel recommended. The journal studied more than 200 guidelines held in the U.S. National Guideline Clearinghouse in 2004. Of the 90 guidelines that contained details about individual authors' conflicts of interest, only 31 had no industry influence. The primary types of conflict included participating in industry-sponsored seminars and owning stock in companies being considered (10% of panels had at least one member in this category). Forty-nine percent of guidelines did not contain any information about panelists' conflicts of interest.

It has been estimated that as many as 90% of authors of clinical practice guidelines, whether or not they purport to represent purely evidence-based practice, report some financial relationship with a for-profit corporation (Warner & Roberts, 2004). Similar results were reported in a study of 789 papers in 14 medical journals that found that one third of the first authors had a financial conflict of interest (Warner & Roberts, 2004). Estimates of the number of practice guideline panelists with conflicts of interest are undoubtedly low since they rely on self-disclosure and a substantial number do not provide any information about conflict of interest. According to the Center for Science in the Public Interest's Integrity in Science Project, "it is usually the journals and supplements that rely heavily on industry advertising that are least likely to have good disclosure policies" (Reichardt, 2005, p. 1070). Interestingly, most authors of clinical practice guidelines are three times as likely to think that their coauthors' opinions are influenced by their relationship with industry as they are to think that such factors influence their own opinions (Warner & Roberts, 2004).

Some treatment guidelines involve data largely from industry-financed studies that are supported, somewhat like a celebrity endorsement, by leaders in the field, many of whom have a financial relationship with the manufacturer of the product being tested (Healy & Thase, 2003). As a result, some symposia and reports start to sound like infomercials. One of the darker views of this process is proposed by David Healy, who says that "journal editors seem to be the fall guys who, equipped with the shovels of conflict of interest statements and the brooms of authorship declarations, are expected to clean out the Augean stables of an increasingly compromised academic literature" (Healy & Thase, 2003, p. 389). To illustrate physicians' ability to deny the impact of marketing efforts, Healy advises: "Wait for psychiatrists coming out of the exhibition halls laden with pens, mugs, kites and CDs, in a relaxed frame of mind having had their massage done or their portrait painted and ask: Does this not influence you? Our answer invariably is: No. How could this have much effect on us—we follow the evidence" (Healy and Thase, 2003, p. 388).

A remarkable example of drug company involvement in practice guidelines was the development of clinical guidelines for treating AIDS. A group of experts was convened by Ortho Biotech, which funded the meeting that produced the guidelines. All six members of the panel had been paid by Ortho for consulting or lecturing. The guidelines, which were published in *Clinical Infectious Disease* in 2004, recommended epoetin alpha, a drug marketed by Ortho Biotech, for treating anemia. According to Drummond Rennie, deputy editor of *JAMA*, "drug company sponsors see guideline-issuing bodies as perfect places to exert influence. The practice stinks" (Reichardt, 2005, p. 1070).

One problem in recruiting more neutral panelists is that most of the prominent experts in a particular area are recruited by drug companies for seminars and research. One suggested solution is to ask experts with drug company ties to present data to panels made up of neutral experts skilled at examining medical data who do not have such affiliations. However, there may not be enough neutral experts to achieve this goal. For example, the American Diabetes Association estimates that three fourths of its members who are qualified to write guidelines have industry links (Reichardt, 2005). The figure is undoubtedly even higher in psychiatry.

Industry has an impact on the kinds of practice guidelines that are discussed in Chapter 7 through the design and conduct of many of the studies on which the guidelines are based, and through its relationships with the experts who interpret the data and construct the guidelines. Even if such influences could be completely eliminated, however, the scientific clinician will remain critical of the evidence in evidence-based medicine. Whether or not clinical research is sponsored by industry, most good research is designed to address a single question in a limited context and may not be relevant for general clinical practice (March et al., 2005). As described in Chapter 4, this is especially true in psychiatry, where most of the gold-standard randomized controlled trials have been conducted under highly controlled, ideal circumstances that do not apply to real-life practice (Lagomasino, Dwight-Johnson, & Simpson, 2005).

Evidence-based medicine should be based on an integration of data from randomized trials, meta analyses, clinically relevant basic science research, studies of diagnostic tests and prognostic markers, and studies of the efficacy and safety of therapeutic, rehabilitative, and preventive regimens (Feinstein & Horwitz, 1997). In reality, however, most evidence-based recommendations are based on randomized controlled trials and on meta analyses (described in the next chapter), which can aggregate data from randomized trials but are still based on the same data.

Most of the randomized trials on which treatment recommendations are based enroll homogeneous groups of patients who are already known to be likely to respond to the treatment being studied (Feinstein & Horwitz, 1997). Important data such as duration and complexity of illness, previous treatment, treatment adherence, comorbidity, social supports, and clinical subgroups are usually ignored. Studies comparing the addition of one treatment to the addition of another treatment in patients who fail to respond completely to an initial intervention are just beginning to emerge in psychiatry—a marked contrast to specialties such as oncology or infectious disease, where combinations of four treatments of one kind are compared to combinations of four other treatments in a different order and genetic and biological markers as well as diagnostic subtypes are correlated with response to each combination.

DIRECT TO CONSUMER MARKETING AND SUPPORT OF ADVOCACY GROUPS

In 1997, the FDA eased restrictions on direct to consumer (DTC) advertising of medical therapies (Karpay, 2005). Since then, expenditures on drug company advertising have increased from $55 million per year in 1991 to more than $3 billion in 2003 (Abramson, 2004; Moynihan & Cassels, 2005). A recent increase in the use of celebrities to market illnesses and their treatment has increased the influence of this medium (Moynihan & Cassels, 2005). The result has been a proliferation of advertisements that induce patients to ask their physicians for specific medications, especially antidepressants and sleeping pills. In fact, of the 50 most intensively publicly marketed drugs in the United States, 18% are psychiatric and neurological medications (Hollon, 2004).

More than 30 years ago Henry Gadsden, the CEO of Merck, told *Fortune* magazine that to address the problem that "the company's potential markets [have] been limited to sick people," he hoped to "make drugs for healthy people" (Moynihan & Cassels, 2005, p. ix). Today, this dream is being realized in a version of DTC marketing that emphasizes that people may have illnesses that require new treatments (Moynihan, Heath, & Henry, 2002). Such marketing efforts often involve a collaboration among pharmaceutical companies, physicians, and consumer groups under the guise of raising public awareness about underdiagnosed, undertreated illnesses, but their primary purpose is to expand markets for new products (Moynihan, et al., 2002). As Moynihan et al. point out, "In many cases the formula is the same: groups and/or campaigns are orchestrated, funded and facilitated by corporate interests, often via their public relationships and marketing infrastructure" (2002, p. 886).

A "practical guide" published in the British magazine *Pharmaceutical Marketing* (Moynihan et al.) stated that its key objectives prior to marketing a new drug for irritable bowel syndrome were to "establish a need" for a new treatment and "create the desire" among prescribers to treat it (2002, p. 888). Through contracts with medical education groups, some companies have been promoting systematic campaigns to establish certain problems as common illness requiring the treatment manufactured by the sponsor of the campaign. The first step is to convene an advisory board consisting of key opinion leaders to help to establish the market among physicians, pharmacists, nurses, and patients. Sometimes, a foundation for the disorder is established that cements relationships among providers, patients, and families with the company and its product.

An interesting example of the creation of a market for a new drug occurred in Australia when the manufacturer of sildenafil (Viagra) published a newspaper advertisement stating that 39% of Australian men visiting general practitioners had erectile dysfunction (Moynihan et al., 2002). The advertisement featured a picture of a couple who appeared to be in their 30s or 40s, but the survey referred to in the ad, and a similar study that was not cited, actually found that the figure included occasional problems with erection, that only 3% of men in their 40s had erectile dysfunction, and that the average age of men with complete erectile dysfunction was 71 (Moynihan et al., 2002). The advertisement referred readers to a group called Impotence Australia that was started by the manufacturer with a grant of $105,000 (U.S. dollars). Some manufacturers have now established educational programs and formal support for advocacy groups that provide materials these groups could not otherwise afford while creating a positive relationship with the sponsor.

Shortly after the drug was approved for the treatment of mania, an advertisement sponsored by the manufacturer of olanzapine showed a woman who is up late and then goes shopping and is apparently being treated for depression, suggesting that the patient's physician has missed the fact that the depression is really bipolar and that anyone who stays up late, paints their kitchen, or spends too much money could be bipolar (Healy, 2006). The ad encourages viewers to go to the "Bipolar Help Center" Web site, which provides a simple test people can take to tell them whether they are bipolar. The Web site goes on to inform readers that bipolar disorder "is often a lifelong illness needing lifelong treatment" and indirectly portrays the manufacturer as a benevolent institution that is purely interested in the welfare of anyone who might be bipolar.

From 1990 to 1995, prescriptions of methylphenidate (Ritalin and others) for children and adolescents increased two and a half times in the United States and an astounding nine times in New South Wales, Australia (Phillips, 2006). One factor in the increasing use of this and other stimulants such as Adderall (a mixture of two amphetamine isomers), as well as of the nonstimulant atomoxetine (Strattera) has been an expanded DTC campaign. While the manufacturer of Strattera sponsored an effective TV commercial that suggested that anyone who experienced the world as noisy or confusing could have attention deficit hyperactivity disorder (ADHD), the manufacturers of Ritalin and Adderall established Web sites with links to their products that included information for teachers as well as parents. The advice to teachers included the directive to "make it clear to [parents] that it is important for them—and their child—to understand and follow the doctor's medical advice about medication and other therapies for ADHD" (Phillips, 2006, p. 183). A number of other manufacturers produced online educational programs for teachers that do not mention specific medications but that reinforce the role of medications in the treatment of ADHD and that establish the manufacturer as a benevolent partner in the identification and treatment of ADHD in school (Phillips, 2006). If a medication were to be used, the sponsor's product presumably would be an early choice.

Industry has recently developed a rapidly growing liaison with potential consumers by providing educational materials and financial support for advocacy groups that is beginning to seem proportional to the support offered for professional societies. The national survey of patient attitudes toward their treatment described later in this book by the Depression and Bipolar Support Alliance (Alliance, 2006) was supported by Wyeth Pharmaceuticals, and events by other support and advocacy groups have been able to rely on industry support for facilities, materials, and dinners, much as the APA has been able to do over the years. In the fiscal year ending in June 2005, one fifth of the total revenue to the ADHD advocacy group CHADD (Children and Adults with Attention Deficit/Hyperactivity Disorder) came from the pharmaceutical industry (Phillips, 2006).

Support of advocacy groups usually does not come with a specific commercial for a particular product. While providing a definite service to the community and to practitioners, such activities create the same sense of gratitude and the kind of close alliance that can also blur the boundary among education, advocacy, and marketing. The medical director of the Association of the British Pharmaceutical Industry asserted that through DTC activities industry puts evidence-based medicine into practice, and that a given company cannot be criticized for its DTC activity because increasing the market for one product also increases the market for its competitors (Tiner, 2002). Whether or not the benefits of industry sponsorship outweigh the potential undermining of the neutrality of the organization, it is important for participants to be aware of the marketing dimension of the relationship.

One potential impact of DTC marketing is that a 30-second sound bite can present information so definitively that patients end up feeling that the medication being advertised is the best treatment for their condition. This makes it more difficult for the physician to discuss alternative treatments and obtain informed consent. What physician has the credibility of a movie star or a figure on national television? For their part, physicians, who are increasingly pressed for time, when given a choice between helping the patient understand the range of treatment options or spending a minute acceding to the patient's request and writing a prescription that probably makes sense anyway, will probably write the requested prescription (Karpay, 2005).

Another outcome of marketing to patients and prescribers is the increasing use of pharmacological approaches in situations in which the indications may be unclear or even absent. In 2002, 9 out of 10 children treated by a child psychiatrist were taking one or more psychotropic medications, despite evidence that in some situations (e.g., childhood depression), published and unpublished studies demonstrated unreliable effectiveness (Diller, 2005) or even a risk or increasing suicidal thoughts in some patients, possibly those with missed bipolar depression (Hammad, Langhren, & Racoosin, 2006). Lawrence Diller, who attended the 2004 FDA hearings on risks of SSRIs in children, learned that eight negative studies of SSRIs in children were not published because the manufacturers were under no legal obligation to publicize them and doing so would have been contrary to the interests of their stockholders (Diller, 2005). Diller said that his experience led him to feel that "academic medicine . . . was being corrupted by its growing dependency on drug company funding. As a front-line physician having to make daily decisions about whom to medicate, I find that I have lost faith in my academic colleagues to give me unbiased advice" (2005, p. 29).

What about the marketing of treatments for conditions that are not necessarily illnesses? The comedian Chris Rock says that after rejecting one ad after another for one kind of distress or another, he finally heard one that said, "Do you go to sleep at night and wake up in the morning?" He jumped up immediately and exclaimed, "I've got that!" Anyone who has seen the rash of advertisements for new hypnotic agents knows that Rock's reaction was not facetious. The advertisements, which feature people sleeping peacefully, make it look like the nights of interrupted sleep that almost everyone experiences are evidence of illness and that the right medication can eliminate the disruptions of everyday life. Yet even true insomnia is more effectively treated with cognitive and behavioral treatments than with sleeping pills, and these kinds of promotions make it easier for people to reach for a medication for any problem they encounter, and for physicians to prescribe a medication before considering resources patients have within themselves to solve the problem. It is not necessary for this kind of marketing to stop, but anyone treating patients should be aware of its impact on patients' orientation toward their conditions.

Research Design 101

2

Most of us do not have the time or expertise to read through every study that comes out. If we do not rely simply on what industry or the experts tell us, we read the abstract and possibly the last few sentences without really knowing whether the conclusions are justified by the results. We have trusted the reviewers to decide for us whether the study is valid, but as the previous chapter demonstrated, reviewers and journals can have the same blind spots as everyone else. Ultimately, our patients depend on us to evaluate the research on which we base our treatment decisions. This chapter provides a structure for evaluating such research. You may want to read it in its entirety now, or you may prefer just to read sections that apply to a research report you want to evaluate.

New treatments are usually developed because they resemble a known effective treatment or because clinicians notice a new effect of an existing treatment; less frequently, a new therapy is based on a theoretical model that might or might not be correct. The classic example of the latter is the development of electroconvulsive therapy (ECT). Based on the mistaken impression that schizophrenia and epilepsy did not occur together, it seemed logical that inducing seizures might be a treatment for schizophrenia. The first few patients treated with convulsions induced by camphor did improve dramatically, although in retrospect they probably had catatonia, and the use of an electrical stimulus to induce seizures more predictably was rewarded with the Nobel Prize. It is now known that epilepsy does not protect against schizophrenia—indeed, epilepsy can cause a schizophrenia-like psychosis. In addition, ECT is primarily a treatment for mood disorders, not schizophrenia.

Many journals publish articles about one or a series of patients who seemed to benefit from open treatment with a new medication. These reports provide a reason to study the potential utility of the new treatment formally, but they do not prove that it works. To address that possibility, it is necessary to do a controlled clinical trial in which patients are randomly assigned to the new treatment or to a comparison treatment. Because of the high placebo response rate in major depressive, anxiety, and even bipolar disorders, one comparator is usually a placebo. A placebo comparison should not be as necessary for disorders with a low rate of spontaneous improvement or response to placebo, such as schizophrenia, but the FDA still requires a placebo arm in clinical trials performed to obtain approval of a new drug. Even without a placebo, however, it is necessary to compare a new treatment to an established treatment and to assess improvement blind to the treatment condition.

A scientific study should test a hypothesis or, put another way, it should attempt to disprove a null hypothesis. The null hypothesis is the opposite of the hypothesis the researcher hopes is true. In a study of an antidepressant in major depression, for example, the null hypothesis would be that there will be no difference in depression rating scale scores between patients treated with an antidepressant and those receiving a placebo. Most moderately sized studies examine a single or at most two primary outcomes. A study may add a number of secondary outcome measures such as response of subgroups, social functioning, correlations of response with blood levels, or side effects, but the study is not designed to test hypotheses related to these factors, and the only valid use of secondary findings is to generate new hypotheses to be tested in additional studies. This is an extremely important point to consider when evaluating new research since many of the articles that are published today draw conclusions from secondary measures that should not be used to prove anything.

For example, a good deal of anxiety was aroused by the finding introduced on page 18 that antidepressants increase suicidality in children and adolescents. The study that led to this conclusion (Hammad et al., 2006) was a reanalysis of data from 24 trials lasting 4 to 16 weeks in 4,582 children and adolescents prescribed

fluoxetine, sertraline, paroxetine, fluvoxamine, citalopram, bupro-
pion, venlafaxine, nefazodone, and mirtazapine for major depression (16 trials), obsessive compulsive disorder (4 trials), general-
ized anxiety disorder (2 trials), and social anxiety disorder (1
trial). One of the depression trials was an NIMH-funded multicenter randomized trial, while the rest were sponsored by the
manufacturer in order to obtain FDA approval for a pediatric
indication. All of the studies were designed to test the hypothesis that the antidepressant was better than placebo in reducing
symptoms. As secondary measures, the studies collected spontaneous reports of adverse events that included suicidal thoughts
and attempts, and each study used a rating scale that had a question about suicidal thoughts.

Aggregating the data from all the studies retrospectively, the
FDA authors defined *suicidality* as new or increased suicidal
thoughts, preparation for a suicide attempt, or an actual suicide
attempt. No suicides occurred in any of the trials, four trials had
no ideation or attempts, and only one trial (the NIMH study)
had a statistically significant increased risk of suicidality with
the antidepressant compared to placebo. However, pooling data
from all the trials with the more conservative model—suicidality
with antidepressants—was about 1.75 as likely as with placebo
for all patients and 1.66 times as likely for patients in major depression trials. This finding led to the addition of a warning to
the package insert of all antidepressants that these medicines
could increase suicide risk in children and adolescents. As one
result of the new warning, pediatricians, who provide the bulk
of psychotropic medication prescriptions for children, are now
reluctant to prescribe antidepressants for any reason to these
patients.

One of the biggest problems with the conclusion of the FDA
analysis is that each of the studies used different patient populations, different assessments, and different durations of treatment, and none of them were designed to determine the effect
of the medication on suicidal intention; to do so would have required more comprehensive questioning of patients and their
families using more detailed suicide rating instruments, as well
as longer follow-up. The relative duration of exposure was the

same for antidepressants and placebos, but if patients who were more likely to have suicidal thoughts dropped out of the placebo group sooner than the antidepressant group because they did not notice any benefit, it might have made placebo appear less likely to be associated with suicidality. Even if *suicidality* as defined by the FDA group actually was a measure of risk of suicide or some other bad outcome, the most that could be concluded is that a better measure of the risk should be devised so that a study could be designed specifically to test the risk of suicidality and its association with actual suicide.

The first decision in designing a clinical trial, therefore, is the condition to be studied. It may seem obvious that the investigator will compare treatments in major depression, panic disorder, bipolar disorder, or whatever condition is of interest, but the disorders most of us treat are not so straightforward. If depressed patients who use substances are included, they may have a lower treatment response and it may be harder to determine whether a new antidepressant works for the disorder, but if substance users are excluded, it will not be possible to tell whether the large number of depressed patients who use substances will be likely to benefit. In either case, how narrowly should the disorder under study be defined? Some patients with a disorder such as major depression or schizophrenia have an early onset and some have a late onset; some have severe symptoms and some have mild symptoms; some patients have multiple recurrences and others just a few; some have had traumatic experiences and others have not; some have psychotic or dissociative symptoms and others do not. These patients have different courses and probably different responses to the same treatment.

The reason why no treatment is universally effective is that some diagnostic subtypes may have a good response and others do not. If a homogeneous sample that is likely to respond to the treatment is chosen (e.g., mild to moderate nonpsychotic unipolar depression for an SSRI trial), it will not be scientifically possible to generalize to all depressed patients, while if the treatment does not work it will remain unknown whether it might be more effective in another subtype. A study of a more heterogeneous sample will require a much larger number of subjects to determine who responds to the treatment and who does not. The results will be more useful, however, in everyday practice since most specialists do not see the kinds of uncomplicated patients who are used as subjects in most trials designed to demonstrate efficacy of treatment to be submitted to the FDA.

WHAT DOES RESEARCH MEASURE?

While suicide is a discrete event, differences of opinion about the meaning of *suicidality* underscore the importance of defining the outcome measure of a study as precisely as possible. Many psychiatric studies have focused on symptom reduction, usually measured by changes on a validated rating scale such as the HDRS (or HAM-D), the Young Mania Rating Scale (YMRS), or the Positive and Negative Symptom Scale (PANSS) for schizophrenia, which are completed by an interviewer, or the Beck Depression Inventory (BDI), which is completed by the patient. The Clinical Global Impression (CGI) scale is used in many clinical trials to represent the clinician's overall impression of how ill the patient is at baseline and whether the patient is better, worse, or the same with treatment.

Average changes in rating scale scores in a large group of subjects are just that—the average of scores of patients who improved, those who were unchanged, and those who got worse. To obtain an estimate of the number of patients who actually benefited, rates of response and remission are computed. In depression studies, response, a measure of whether the patient is better, is commonly defined as at least a 50% reduction in depression rating scale scores. Remission (i.e., the patient is well) is technically defined as minimal or no symptoms and the patient no longer meeting criteria for a major depressive episode, but in most antidepressant trials remission is defined as an HDRS score of 7 or less and a CGI rating of improved or very much improved—close, but not exactly the same thing. Because patients with schizophrenia do not usually have the same expectation of improvement, response is usually arbitrarily defined in studies of this disorder as a 30% or greater reduction of symptom rating scale scores.

To approve a new medication, the FDA only requires evidence of a statistically significantly greater rate of response with the new medication than with a placebo. However, patients who have just had a response are not well. They continue to be symptomatic, their symptoms interfering with their functioning. So far, the FDA has not required that a new treatment demonstrate improved functioning in important roles, productivity, or even enjoyment of life. However, improvement in functioning often lags behind symptomatic improvement, and in view of the traditional definition of a psychiatric disorder as consisting both of symptoms and impaired functioning, patients with continued impairment are still ill. Even more important, residual psychosocial impairment increases the risk of major symptomatic relapse.

Just as the study of an oncology drug should demonstrate that the drug gets rid of residual cancer cells and eliminates residual evidence of pathophysiology in addition to shrinking tumors, it has become increasingly apparent that to assess the true effect of a psychiatric treatment it is necessary to go beyond specific symptoms and a broad impression of whether the patient is functioning and feeling better. In the 1990s, drug companies began to introduce quality of life scales in clinical trials, but fewer than 10% of studies report the results (Healy, 1999), mainly if the study is designed to gain a competitive advantage over other products in the class.

A standard measure of quality of life is the quality-adjusted life year (QALY), which considers the quantity and quality of life generated by an intervention that compares the relative merits of different treatments. A cost of $50,000 per QALY is accepted as a cost-effective use of resources (Lagomasino et al., 2005). Survival curves plot a measure of survival as a function of time. Obviously, remaining alive is an easily replicable outcome but it is rarely used in psychiatry studies. More common survival measures include time to relapse, hospitalization, institution of additional treatment, suicide attempt, or withdrawal from the study. The latter measure—survival in the study—was the primary measure in the well-publicized trial comparing atypical antipsychotic drugs and the neuroleptic perphenazine described on pp. 88–90.

TYPES OF STUDIES

Studies of new treatments fall into two broad categories. Efficacy studies test whether a treatment works, usually compared with a placebo, for people who keep taking it under ideal conditions with minimal complications. Industry-sponsored trials are paradigms of the efficacy study, using homogeneous samples and intensive assessment to address one or two primary outcomes (March et al., 2005), usually in patients who are much more likely to adhere to treatment than patients in actual practice (Lagomasino et al., 2005). This approach maximizes sensitivity for a positive result in a comparison of an active treatment and a placebo on the primary outcome measure (usually changes on a symptom rating scale) with the smallest possible sample size. Efficacy studies utilize extensive quality assurance measures such as face-to-face training, site visits, and extensive chart reviews that may limit the size of the study because they take so much time and effort (March et al., 2005). Some efficacy studies have one or more substudies that examine pharmacokinetics, genetics, or some other factor that requires more intensive and expensive assessment but cannot be used to draw conclusions, unless the factor in the substudy was included in an a priori hypothesis.

Effectiveness studies test the hypothesis that a treatment really works in the large group of people for whom it is prescribed. Since patients who stop the medication early will not benefit from it, an assessment of effectiveness requires considering in the analysis whether they keep taking it. The focus of an effectiveness trial is on gathering information that will be of most interest to clinicians and decision makers. This goal is addressed by enrolling somewhat more heterogeneous samples from a large group of practices and by assessing a wider range of primary outcomes (March et al., 2005). Effectiveness trials usually compare two or more active treatments, including nonpharmacologic treatments (Lagomasino et al., 2005). Such trials include a range of outcomes such as functioning, quality of life, and cost, which are more relevant to patients than in efficacy trials (Lagomasino et al., 2005). Like efficacy trials, effectiveness trials usually enroll hundreds of patients, are conducted in academic or private research centers, and are able to detect a difference between treatment arms of about 20%. Recent NIMH-sponsored studies such as the Systematic Treatment Enhancement Program for Bipolar Disorder (STEP-BD) study combine efficacy (involving intensive assessments) and effectiveness (broad sample) elements.

Randomized clinical trials (RCTs) are considered the gold standard in all branches of medicine. In these studies, which may be designed as efficacy or effectiveness trials, patients are randomly assigned to one or more active treatments or a placebo. Outcome raters, those administering the treatment, and patients are all blind to the group to which the patient was assigned. However, while the study may show clearly that one treatment is on average superior to placebo or better than another treatment, it does not say which outcome is more likely in a given patient (Horwitz, 1995). The true scientific value of a randomized clinical trial is to resolve significant uncertainty about the value of one treatment compared to another, not to prove that treatments are equivalent (Djulbegovic et al., 2000). However, as is discussed a little later, most industry-sponsored trials use the RCT method to do just that.

The cohort study uses a naturalistic method in patients who are already being treated (Levine et al., 1994). This method identifies two groups of patients who are matched for relevant variables and follows them prospectively. It is primarily useful when patients cannot be randomly assigned but an important clinical question must be answered, especially in studies of harmful events such as exposure to toxins or serious adverse effects of treatments.

Practical clinical trials compare clinically important interventions in a diverse population that is more representative of clinical practice than effectiveness or efficacy trials. These studies include heterogeneous practice settings that represent clinical practice and measure a broad range of clinically relevant health outcomes (March et al., 2005). Practical clinical trials have eight defining principles (March et al., 2005):

- The questions asked are simple, clinically relevant, and of substantial health importance. For example, does a given treatment that can be readily used in practice alter important outcomes of depression?

- The studies are performed in clinical practice settings. The study population must be sufficiently heterogeneous and studied in enough clinical practice settings to permit generalization.
- Study power (i.e., the number of subjects enrolled given the likely difference between groups) is sufficient to identify small to moderate effects of around 2.5–10%. These studies are usually larger and simpler than other studies, enrolling thousands of patients in hundreds of locations, a number that is rare in psychotropic studies. Practical clinical trials are more likely than other studies to involve head-to-head comparisons of treatments with clinically relevant, if modest, differences.
- Patients are randomized to prevent selection bias.
- The study question represents an important area of clinical uncertainty. The study is not worth conducting if there is already a substantial empirical basis for preferring one treatment over another. Only true uncertainty about whether one treatment is better than another (or placebo) really justifies enrolling patients in a randomized trial.
- Outcomes are simple and clinically relevant. Unambiguous, readily detectable endpoints are used that can be recognized easily by clinicians and/or patients and represent living longer, feeling better, functioning better, spending less money, and other meaningful outcomes. Outcome measures are easy to administer and score objectively.
- Assessments and treatments reflect best real life clinical practice and not some idealized approach.
- Subject and researcher burden are minimized. It should be possible to complete the trial in a timely manner by using simple methods and a relatively small number of data elements. Otherwise, a study involving thousands of patients and a variety of investigators will be difficult to interpret.

Practical clinical trials funded by federal sources are common for heart disease and cancer (March et al., 2005). For example, the Virtual Coordinating Center for Global Cardiovascular Research network has conducted 15 thrombolytic trials in more than 150,000 patients at 3,000 sites in 50 countries, and more than 95% of American children with cancer are treated at the 500 centers participating in the NCI-funded Children's Oncology Group network (March et al., 2005). Similarly, because Type I antiarrhythmics suppress ventricular premature beats, it seemed logical to assume that they would reduce mortality after myocardial infarction (M.I.). The Cardiac Arrhythmia Suppression Trials (CAST) looked at whether this would be the case in a practical clinical trial model and found that the Type I antiarrhythmics actually increased mortality by 250%, whereas the newer Type III antiarrhythmics did reduce mortality (March et al., 2005). Industry is not likely to fund these kinds of practical clinical trials that can provide data important to public health or clinical standards if such trials could put profits at risk (March et al., 2005).

A single RCT cannot prove that a specific treatment is effective or that it is superior to anything else. This is especially true in psychiatry, where studies tend to be smaller than in other specialties. Meta-analysis has emerged as a method of combining the results of multiple RCTs. Meta-analysis is now used frequently to draw conclusions about the benefits of one treatment relative to one or more other treatments. This approach uses a set of procedures to combine the results of different studies, increasing the statistical power to detect moderate-sized effects and reconciling conflicting results (Horwitz, 1995). However, the methodology of psychiatric studies that are combined with meta-analysis may be so different that combining them is not justified. Furthermore, a meta-analysis of trials that are flawed will be flawed itself (Feinstein, 1995). Estimations of treatment differences are more precise in a 2,000-subject parallel group practical clinical trial than a meta-analysis of 10 underpowered 200-subject efficacy trials (March et al., 2005), just as combining inadequate doses of two antidepressants does not necessarily equal a therapeutic dose of one of them.

ANALYZING DATA

The way in which the results of a study are analyzed depends on the trial design. For example, the best way to assess efficacy is to use a completer analysis. Since the question being asked is whether the treatment is inherently efficacious, results are analyzed for subjects who continue the treatment at a sufficient dose long enough for it to work, which in most psychiatry studies is 1 to 3 months. If the assumption is that a treatment will not be as useful if patients do not take it long enough for an effect to become manifest, an intent-to-treat model with the last observation carried forward (LOCF) is used. In this model, the last result available from all patients who take at least one dose of a medication is considered the final value. Since nonadherence and other prognostic factors are supposedly equally distributed in both groups, the medication is considered ineffective in patients who stop it early because of side effects or other problems with the treatment.

The LOCF method is thought to reflect real-life outcomes because it considers whether patients keep taking the medication, but it ignores effects in patients who do continue to take the medication (Feinstein & Horwitz, 1997). For example, in randomized trials SSRIs appeared to be at least as effective as tricyclic antidepressants such as imipramine, because imipramine is not as well tolerated and is more likely to be discontinued early, but for more severely depressed patients who are more motivated to continue it until it works, imipramine may be more helpful. At the same time, the completer analysis misses the impact of adherence to treatment. The wise clinician therefore looks for both results.

Even though the LOCF method is accepted by the FDA, it has significant flaws. Average dropout rates of 37% have been reported in antidepressant studies, 50–64% in antipsychotic studies, and 30% in studies of the treatment of geriatric depression (Leon et al., 2006). The assumption that the last available measure represents how all of these subjects would have done in the long run is not supported by any actual data (Leon et al., 2006). The other assumption on which LOCF rests, namely, that because patients who dropped out were similar in age and symptom severity to those who remained in the study they would not have had a different outcome, is also not necessarily correct. Dropping out of a study is not a random phenomenon, and there is usually not enough information about dropouts and their eventual outcomes to know how closely our patients resemble them and whether our patients are therefore equally likely to drop out of the same treatment.

There are a number of statistical methods that can correct for the effect on the overall outcome of patients who did not remain in the study (Leon et al., 2006). For example, results from dropouts can be analyzed according to how symptomatic they were when they withdrew. It is also possible to plot the trajectory of response in patients who have had more than one measure, and to analyze results differently for patients who remained in the study for varying periods of time. In some analyses, several possible outcomes are computed for each subject, and the possibilities are averaged for an expected outcome. As most Phase III studies do not do any of these corrections, we have an additional level of uncertainty about the outcome in all patients who start the treatment.

THE TERMINOLOGY OF STATISTICS

When we read research studies, symposia, and even industry brochures, we come across a host of statistical terms, most of which we have not seen since medical school. The following discussion defines the terms and concepts that are most important in understanding modern psychiatric research (Beasley et al., 1991; Guyatt, Sackett, & Cook, 1994; Kraemer & Kupfer, 2006; Lagomasino et al., 2005; Motulsky, 1995).

All clinical populations are heterogeneous, especially in psychiatry. Any study that reports results for all subjects that are very close to each other—for example, all patients improved to the same degree—is difficult to believe unless subjects were selected very carefully prior to the study for exactly the same characteristics. As a result, well-conducted and believable studies report a range of results. The standard deviation (SD) measures the scatter of the data. The standard error of the mean (SEM), calculated as $SD/\sqrt{N}$, measures how close the sample mean is to the mean in the larger population from which the sample is drawn, such as all patients with major depressive disorder or schizophrenia. Many investigators like to use the SEM because it is usually smaller than the SD and can be represented on a graph with easily read range-of-value horizontal lines across a bar graph. However, the SEM is not a direct measure of scatter of the data, so it is important not to mistake SEM bars in a graph for variability of the results.

Any study that is designed to disprove a null hypothesis has to have a sufficient number of subjects to produce significant results. This decision is based on a power analysis. A power analysis tells the experimenter how likely it is that an important difference between groups will be found and is based on the expected variability of the data. A study felt to have a probability greater than around 80% of demonstrating a significant difference between treatments is generally considered adequately powered. If there is likely to be a large range of results, it will be necessary to include more patients in each group to show that any difference between the groups is not accidental. For this reason, a power analysis depends on the SD of the data, which can often be obtained from other observations of similar patients. All studies have little power to detect small differences and great power to detect substantial differences; increasing the sample size increases the power.

After analyzing data, the researcher has to decide whether the results are statistically significant. Two methods are commonly used to compare groups of patients. The p value is calculated as the probability of getting a difference as large as or larger than the one that would be observed if the null hypothesis were correct. The p value tells us how sure we are that there is a real difference between populations and that the difference is not coincidental.

A p value of 0.05 means that the observed difference will occur by chance 5% of the time. Stated differently, if the same experiment is conducted 100 times, the results in the experiment will be obtained by chance in 5 of them. However, this does not mean that there is a 95% chance that the difference between groups is real; it just means that if the null hypothesis is true, 95% of experiments would yield a difference smaller than the observed difference and 5% would yield a difference greater than the observed difference. The p value only indicates how rarely a difference would be observed that is greater than or the same as the observed one if the null hypothesis is true. It is a matter of interpretation whether this is so unlikely that the null hypothesis can be discarded. In other words, a significant p value tells us that the result is likely not to be random, but it provides no information about how large or important the result is.

How many times are lower p values (e.g., $p < 0.0001$) called "highly significant," presumably more so than $p < 0.05$? Investigators may interpret their findings in this manner, but statisticians do not agree (Kraemer & Kupfer, 2006; Motulsky, 1995). Once a decision is made about the threshold for statistical significance, the results are either significant or not significant; the difference from the a priori level of significance (described a few paragraphs from here) does not matter. The only meaning of the degree of difference from the threshold of significance is that if the observed p is very close to that value, confidence that p meets the threshold may not be as great as it would be if it were substantially lower. So if $p = 0.049$, the chance that it is certainly less than 0.05 is not as great as it would be if $p = 0.001$. Conversely, if $p = 0.001$, you cannot infer any more than that it is definitely less than 0.05.

By the same token, a p value that is not significant does not prove that the experimental treatment was not effective. It may mean that the study was not designed to demonstrate a meaningful result. However, when an article reports "a significant trend" where p is somewhere between 0.05 and 0.1 or even higher, the most that can be said is that the finding may be worth a separate study. The reader should ignore any attempt to go on to discuss the result as if it were actually statistically significant. Statistically significant just means statistically significant. A trend is a finding that is not statistically significant but may be worth investigating later. There is no such thing as a significant trend.

The result of any clinical trial is called a point estimate because the true value lies somewhere around, but not exactly at, that value. The neighborhood in which the true effect is likely to lie is indicated by the confidence interval (CI). The 95% CI is the range that includes the true result 95% of the time, while the true result is outside this range only 5% of the time. This range is analogous to the conventional level of statistical significance of $p < 0.05$. You can therefore be 95% sure that the average difference between populations is within the 95% CI. In general, if the 95% CI includes the null hypothesis (in other words, if the value that would indicate no difference between the experimental treatment and a placebo is within that range), p is greater than 0.05 and the results are not significant. The more scattered the results, the wider the CI. The larger the study, the narrower the CI and the closer the result is to the true difference between treatments or between active treatments and placebo.

To avoid retrospectively fitting data to the hypothesis rather than the other way around, researchers decide in advance the threshold level at which the results will be considered statistically significant. By tradition, the threshold (referred to as α) for this decision is usually set arbitrarily at a p value of 0.05 or its equivalent (Motulsky, 1995). While this cutoff is taken as gospel by many readers, it is actually completely arbitrary. In reality, α should be determined based on the purpose of the study and the number and kind of statistical tests that will be performed. Setting α very low reduces the chance of making a Type I error or "statistical false positive," in which an apparently significant result is not really significant. However, a low α will increase the chance of a Type II error, in which a result that really is statistically significant is rejected as not significant—in other words, a false negative.

The decision where to set α therefore depends on the potential consequences of Type I and Type II errors, which depends on the reason for the study. For example (Motulsky, 1995), in a Phase III clinical trial of a drug for which other effective therapies exist (e.g., an antidepressant for nonpsychotic depression or an antipsychotic drug for mania), the consequence of a Type I error would be that an ineffective drug would appear to work and would be marketed, resulting in patients being treated with a drug (and probably an expensive one) that does not really work when more effective drugs are already on the market. A Type II error would lead to rejecting a good medication, but other effective treatments would be available. In this situation, from a scientific standpoint the level of significance might be set at 0.01 because a Type I error would be less harmful than a Type II error, while from a marketing standpoint α might be set at 0.05 to maximize the chance that the new product will look significantly better than placebo. Conversely, in a Phase III study of a treatment for a disease for which there are no clearly effective treatments such as bipolar depression, science might dictate setting a higher α because a Type II error would not hurt patients any more than they would be hurt by having no treatment at all, whereas a Type I error might lead to abandonment of a drug that might turn out to be useful when nothing better is on the market.

Many industry-sponsored studies examine multiple outcomes at the same time, setting α at 0.05. However, when several null hypotheses are tested at the same time, the chance of a spurious significant result increases. Consider a study that examines whether a new mood stabilizer is better than an existing medication in reducing depression scores, decreasing mania scores, and having fewer sedative side effects. If the three independent null hypotheses (no difference in improvement of depression or mania or in side effects) are tested at the same time using $\alpha = 0.05$, there is a 14% likelihood of observing one or more significant p value (i.e., $p < 0.05$) even if all three null hypotheses are true (Motulsky, 1995). A rule of thumb for figuring out whether results are really statistically significant for 10 or fewer comparisons is to divide 0.05 by the number of comparisons. For example, to be confident that any of the results is really significant at a level equivalent to $p < 0.05$ in the case of the mood stabilizer study, the threshold for significance should be decreased from 0.05 to 0.017 (0.05/3). If seven hypotheses were being tested in the same study, the threshold should be $0.05/7 = 0.0071$. If 100 independent null hypotheses are tested, there is a 99% chance of obtaining at least one spurious significant p value, and you would not know which of the results was invalid.

Chapter 5 describes instances in which a statistically significant result is reported for statistical tests done on multiple variables at the same time (the CATIE [Clinical Antipsychotic Trials of Intervention Effectiveness] study is one such example). Then, a correction is made for the multiple comparisons, after which some or all of the results are no longer significant. In such reports, it is important not to go with first impressions; namely, that the result is significant, when it really is not. Without reading such a report carefully, it is easy to be deceived into thinking that the results were significant. This issue is magnified when retrospective analyses are done once a study is completed (data dredging). Data dredging can be useful in uncovering trends that are worth making into hypotheses to be tested prospectively. There is no justification for using such results to draw conclusions about the treatment being tested. Yet it is not uncommon to see a report of a Phase III study in which the primary result was marginally significant or insignificant, but one or more findings that emerged as all the other data were analyzed are reported as statistically significant, often without even correcting for multiple comparisons. Such results might be worth a somewhat interested shrug, but not much more.

A binary difference between one treatment and another (i.e., the experimental treatment is or is not better) can be effectively presented as an odds ratio (OR). The OR is defined as the probability that an event will occur (e.g., that an antidepressant will be superior to a placebo) divided by the probability that it will not occur, or the ratio of the odds of improvement with the study drug versus the odds of improvement with placebo or another treatment. In contrast, the probability an event will occur is the fraction of times it is expected in a given number of trials. Probabilities range from 0 to 1; odds can be 0 or any positive number. For example, the probability of a flipped coin landing on heads is 50%; the odds of the same outcome is $50:50 = 1$. If the probability is 0.75, the odds are $0.75:0.25 = 3$. If the odds of hallucinations are 0.19 with an antipsychotic drug and 0.39 with placebo, the OR is $0.19/0.39 = 0.49$, indicating that the odds of hallucinations in patients taking an antipsychotic is half that with placebo. Because values beyond the upper and lower boundaries of the 95% CI are very unlikely to represent the true result, when the 95% CI of an OR includes 1, the experimental treatment is not likely to be truly different from the control. ORs are essential when analyzing retrospective case control studies but not prospective, cross-sectional, or experimental studies.

The relative risk (RR), or the ratio of the risk of illness or symptoms in patients on the new treatment relative to controls (risk with the therapy divided by risk without therapy), is another way of looking at the difference between treatments. An RR between 0 and 1 signifies that the risk decreases with treatment. For example, if 16% of patients treated with an antidepressant are still depressed after 8 weeks but 28% of those treated with placebo are still depressed, the relative risk is 16% / 28% = 0.57. In other words, patients treated with the antidepressant are 57% as likely as those getting placebo to still be depressed. An RR greater than 1 indicates that the risk increases with the study treatment. When the RR = 1, the risk is the same whether or not the subject got the treatment or was exposed to the risk factor. Our confidence that the RR is reliable is measured by the CI, which, if it includes 1, suggests that the treatment is not likely to be significantly different from the comparison.

Absolute risk reduction (risk difference) is the risk of illness without the experimental therapy minus the risk with the therapy. Relative risk reduction (RRR) is defined as absolute RR divided by the risk without the new therapy times 100%. The greater the RRR, the more effective the therapy. For example, in a study of an antidepressant in 100 patients, 20% of the control group did not respond (risk of continued depression without therapy) and 15% of the treatment group did not respond (risk with therapy). In this study, the absolute risk reduction is 0.20 − 0.15, or 0.05. The RR is 0.15/0.20 = 0.75 (i.e., the risk of remaining in the depressed category with the new treatment is 75% that of controls). The RRR is (0.05/0.20) × 100% = 25%, indicating that the new treatment reduced the risk of nonresponse by 25% relative to the rate of nonresponse in controls.

How believable is this estimate? With just 100 patients, the RRR is based on a difference of just 5 patients. In this study, the 95% CI of the RRR is −38% to 59%, so the actual RRR might be 0% (no benefit) or negative (the treatment is harmful). If there were 1,000 patients rather than 100 patients in the study and the same differences occurred, there would be 200 nonresponders in the control group and 150 in the treatment group, so the RRR is still 25%, but the 95% CI is 9–41%, and all possible differences are greater than 0, giving the new treatment more support.

The number needed to treat (NNT) is the reciprocal of the absolute RR, or the number of patients that would have to be treated to prevent one event or produce one result, such as a response of depression. If the patient's risk without treatment is high enough, and the NNT is above a certain threshold, treatment is justified. If the patient's risk without treatment is low and the NNT is above the threshold, treatment would be deferred. The threshold NNT is determined by identifying the target event (e.g., suicide) and the adverse effects caused by treatment. The threshold NNT (i.e., the NNT at which the treatment is worth giving) is determined by assigning relative values to the costs and risks of treating, the costs and risks saved when the target event is prevented, and the adverse events and costs associated with no treatment. For example, beta-blockers reduce the risk of death following M.I. by 25% (RRR). An otherwise healthy patient with a small M.I. and otherwise good health has a risk of death in the first year after M.I. of 1%, and beta-blockers would reduce this by 25% to 0.25% (0.0025). The NNT is 1/0.0025 = 400, so it would be necessary to treat 400 patients to prevent one death. An older patient with multiple risk factors may have a risk of dying in the first year after M.I. of 10%. A 25% RRR produces an absolute RR of 25% of the baseline 10% risk, or 2.5% (0.025). In this case, the NNT = 1/0.025 = 40, so only 40 patients would have to be treated to prevent one death. Like the OR, the NNT is applied to binary outcomes (the treatment does or does not work) and not to continuous variables such as absolute reduction in depression scores.

We will generally accept a higher NNT for a low-risk, cheap, noninvasive intervention with the potential for substantial benefit such as aspirin to reduce the risk of M.I. (NNT = 130). For a safe HIV vaccine, an acceptable NNT might be much higher than that. The NNT for improvement with psychotherapy is only 3.1, but psychotherapy is not used as routinely as aspirin or vaccines because the clinical consequences of not preventing M.I. or AIDS are more profound than the consequences of not reaching a given threshold for benefit from psychotherapy, which in most studies involves being "better off" than without therapy, but not necessarily well (Kraemer & Kupfer, 2006). With more studies of the effectiveness of psychotherapy in producing remission of major mood disorders, the NNT may be somewhat higher but still in a range that would promote scientific clinicians to recommend it as an early intervention.

Statistically significant does not automatically mean clinically significant (Motulsky, 1995). As we have already seen, this is especially true of changes in scores on a single rating scale or response rates—who would be satisfied, for example, with being 50% less depressed and having about as much trouble functioning, or with being 30% less psychotic, even if significantly more patients had this result with the new treatment than with a placebo? A very large study will find that small differences in any outcome, including a meaningful one, are statistically significant, but the difference still may not have major clinical implications. It is therefore important to look for evidence that statistically significant results are clinically meaningful. This should involve more than a statement to the effect that results of a certain magnitude are likely to be clinically important. The investigators should help the reader to understand the clinical implications of the level of improvement, such as with case examples.

A test that can be a little closer to clinical significance is effect size, which indicates the magnitude of the difference between a new treatment and a placebo or an existing treatment. The clinical importance of a finding is inferred by setting an a priori effect size that would be considered meaningful and then looking at how close the effect size in a study comes to that threshold. A common measure of effect size is Cohen's d, which ranges from −1 (the new treatment is clinically worse than the comparator) to 0 (no difference between treatments) to +1 (the new treatment is clinically better). It has been suggested that a d of 0.2 should be considered a small, a d of 0.5 should be considered a medium, and a d of 0.8 should be considered a large effect size, but these judgments might change based on the overall risks and benefits of the treatment (Kraemer & Kupfer, 2006). For example, a small effect size of a relatively risk-free vaccine that prevents a serious disease might make the treatment worth using, while a high effect size in treatment of psychosis of a drug that always causes diabetes might not make the drug worth using as a first-line treatment. As with any result, effect sizes apply to the population that was studied, and not to any individual. This is why the most reliable study to determine whether a particular treatment is right for an individual patient is the *N* of 1 clinical trial (pg. 133). Otherwise, the effect size derived from an RCT is most likely to apply to patients who most closely resemble the patients in the study.

SUBGROUP AND INTERIM ANALYSIS

Subgroup analyses are commonly used to interpret data in a way that was not planned in the original study design. In this method, investigators designate subgroups of subjects by their baseline characteristics and analyze whether the treatment worked differently in these subgroups (Schulz & Grimes, 2005). A frequent motivation for this kind of analysis is a version of data dredging in which an attempt is made to find positive results in some subgroups when the overall result was negative. For example, a study of a mood stabilizer might find no significant difference between a new treatment and an established treatment in the entire sample, but in looking back retrospectively at the results it might appear that the new medication was effective for patients without rapid cycling. The main problem with this approach is that if enough subgroups are tested, false positive results are likely to occur by chance alone (Schulz & Grimes, 2005). As Schulz and Grimes noted, "The answer to a randomized controlled trial that does not confirm one's beliefs is not the conduct of several subanalyses until one can see what one believes. Rather, the answer is to re-examine one's beliefs carefully" (2005, p. 1657).

An example of problems with retrospective subgroup analysis is a study demonstrating that aspirin has a positive effect in preventing death following M.I. ($p < 0.00001$) (Schulz & Grimes, 2005). The authors did a subgroup analysis of the correlation between reduced risk of death and astrological sign that showed that subjects born under signs other than Gemini or Libra were significantly more likely to benefit ($p < 0.00001$), demonstrating that apparently significant but meaningless results will occur randomly in multiple retrospective analyses. It is even more difficult to know what to make of situations in which authors report positive but not negative subgroup analyses. If a subgroup analysis is used, this should be part of the original protocol and all results should be reported (Schulz & Grimes, 2005). The only value of any subgroup analysis that is not specified in advance, no matter how interesting, is to generate hypotheses that can be tested in further studies, as would occur if a prospective study were designed to see if patients without rapid cycling responded to a mood stabilizer after an initial study showed positive results only in the non–rapidly cycling subjects. Any significant effect in a subgroup when there is no overall treatment effect without further research may be provocative, but it has no clinical implications and it should not influence practice standards (Schulz & Grimes, 2005).

Most large studies have a proviso for one or more interim analyses to determine whether evidence is emerging that one of the treatment arms is either so good or so bad that the study should be discontinued. CAST I and II, for example, were designed to compare the ability of different antiarrhythmic drugs to reduce the risk of sudden cardiac death—usually caused by arrhythmia—following M.I. An interim analysis found that the Type Ia antiarrhythmics such as quinidine appeared to increase the risk of sudden death, and the study was discontinued early so that patients taking these medications could be switched to the treatment that was found to reduce the risk of sudden death—beta-blockers. This kind of result is not common in psychiatric studies. Instead, many of these studies are completed but the final sample is much smaller than the sample size that was planned based on a power analysis. The most likely explanation for the study being smaller than originally planned is that more subjects were not enrolled because an interim analysis found that the findings were not likely to be dramatically positive or because it was too expensive to recruit more patients to replace dropouts and the results of early dropouts were considered definitive in a LOCF model (see pp. 50–51). Such an approach is not valid because the results might have been nonsignificant if the trial had been continued at the planned size (Schulz & Grimes, 2005).

HOW TO BE SAFELY
"AHEAD OF THE CURVE"

Industry representatives monitor the prescribing habits of practitioners in their district, and the representatives' status in the company depends in part on whether those habits favor the company's product. Based on data obtained from pharmacies, practitioners are classified according to how soon after a new drug is released they begin prescribing it. Some practitioners like to try new treatments as soon as they are available, while others like to learn more about other people's experience with both positive and negative effects before they prescribe the medication themselves. Some practitioners like to try a new application of a medication as soon as an article is published suggesting that it is helpful, others want to see more data, and some only try a new treatment when it is clearly established.

Drug companies use this information to monitor the effectiveness of their marketing and to decide which practitioners will be most receptive to information about brand-new medications and new indications for their current products. We have even more reason than industry to be aware of the category of provider that best describes us—ahead of the curve, relatively early utilizer of new treatments, waiting for more data, or slow to use new therapies. If we find ourselves on the "cutting edge," whether by temperament or because we have no choice but to try treatments that are not backed by adequate data because nothing else is working, we have a greater responsibility to be aware of the limits of the research that supports these treatments. And there are significant limits to research supporting most combination and high-dose therapies, most treatments for refractory disorders, and most psychotropic medications in children.

As patients become more difficult to treat, more clinicians are moving ahead of the curve and are using treatments based on methodological weaknesses, contradictory findings, patient samples that do not necessarily resemble the patients being treated, and complicated statistical analyses. Clinicians in this setting have a responsibility to synthesize the gaps in data supporting the treatments we recommend and helping the patient to understand how confident it is possible to be about the balance between benefits and risks of the treatments under consideration. After all, it is the patient who has to live with this balance. When patients prefer to delegate the decision completely to the physician, they may be helped to establish a decision-making partnership by clarifying what is frightening about considering the uncertainty of much of our current database.

3

Industry-Sponsored
Clinical Trials

In the 1970s, the pharmaceutical industry began a restructuring process that resulted in a separation of marketing and sales from research. Divisions devoted to research design began to emerge, and industry began actively recruiting the best and the brightest from universities and from government agencies such as NIMH to design their clinical trials. Some companies developed extensive basic science research arms, while others licensed medications developed elsewhere to test and market them.

At one time, industry-sponsored studies were designed by consultants based in academia. In recent years, however, companies have brought research design in-house. Now that they have their own specialists, they use academic consultants drawn from the ranks of investigators with whom they contract to advise them on study design, but the advice may be pro forma (Bodenheimer, 2000). Most manufacturers accept investigator-initiated protocols, but the decision whether to fund these single-site studies depends on whether they fit with marketing directions (Bodenheimer, 2000). Try, for example, asking the manufacturer of a medication that has metabolic side effects to fund a study of mechanisms of weight gain and lipid abnormalities with their product. A competitor might fund a study of that product, but only if it included a comparison with their own product and was designed to show that it did not have the same problem.

While companies are designing their own large trials, these studies have grown so complex that it has been more cost effective to delegate the actual conduct of the research to contract research organizations (CROs) (Bodenheimer, 2000). The CROs then subcontract with both academic and for-profit centers, which recruit subjects and carry out the research. In 2001, there were 1,000 CROs operating around the world with revenues of about $7 billion (Angell, 2005). CROs may monitor the research themselves, or they may subcontract this function to separate site management organizations (SMOs), which provide administrative support for private-practice investigators. Results of the study are drafted by the medical writing division of the company and the principal investigator, who either works for the company or is closely allied with it.

It is both good business and efficient for companies to hire their own principal investigators and for them to rely for additional help on a small, consistent group of independent researchers who share their views of the product. Assembling a group of professional writers to draft articles is no different from the practice of highly productive university research groups that conduct multiple studies at the same time and have a writing staff to help them draft one article after another. The difference is that the combination of absence of true peer review of the research design and delegated research management interacts with a number of other factors to place intermediate steps between generating data and presenting results. Because the study belongs to the company, so do the data; therefore, it seems reasonable to present whatever results seem most appropriate. The limited data that are published may appear in prestigious journals, but conclusions about clinical applications often are not justified because the studies are designed to meet approval criteria for release and marketing and not to test a specific clinical hypothesis independent of these factors.

PHASE I–IV STUDIES

Following animal testing, new drugs are tested in three phases on the way to FDA approval (Angell, 2005). In Phase I, the new molecule is given to a small number of normal subjects to establish safety and to understand drug metabolism. Phase II testing involves a few hundred patients with the illness at which the medication is targeted, mostly to study side effects and optimal dosing. Phase III studies are randomized controlled trials of hundreds (in psychiatry) to thousands (in many other medical specialties) of patients to establish efficacy and safety. The FDA requires demonstration of superiority to placebo in two randomized trials in order to approve a new psychiatric drug.

It is usually necessary to patent a medication before starting clinical testing in order to prevent competitors from developing the same product, but once a patent is obtained the clock on the patent starts ticking and the manufacturer is under tremendous pressure to get the drug to market quickly and earn back its development costs. This factor can have a profound influence on drug development, as occurred when the manufacturer of the reversible monoamine oxidase inhibitor (MAOI) moclobemide (Mannerix), a medication that is in widespread use around the world as a treatment for anxiety and depression because in usual doses it does not have the dietary restrictions necessary with other MAOIs, began conducting Phase III trials in the Unites States. Seeing that the patent would expire not long after the medication might gain approval, and perhaps having used doses in early studies that were too low in order to minimize side effects, the manufacturer withdrew it from development in the United States. Generic companies are not interested in the expense of Phase III testing, so a medication available to clinicians in Canada and South Africa will never be available in this country.

Currently, more medications are subjected to Phase IV (postmarketing) testing to find new uses or unexpected side effects after the drug is released. In addition, the FDA will extend the patent of psychotropic medications that are approved for adults if they undergo Phase IV studies in children. Some Phase IV studies, however, are deceptive. In these studies, large groups of clinicians are recruited to "study" the benefit of a newly released medication in a few of their patients. The "investigators" get a couple of rating scales to fill out, but they receive no training to establish inter-rater reliability (i.e., ratings of the same patient by different observers are similar), and the rating scales are filled out by the same clinician who prescribes the medication. Results of such efforts are of minimal clinical and no scientific value, but the study does accomplish one important goal: the clinician receives a stipend for trying the product and becoming familiar with the medication (Angell, 2005).

In interpreting industry-sponsored Phase III clinical trials, it is important to bear in mind that these studies do not represent research to test an independent hypothesis, but rather, product development to meet regulatory requirements or demonstrate the usefulness of a product (Healy, 1999). The Phase III study therefore has several important differences from independently funded clinical research. For one thing, to demonstrate symptom relief with minimal side effects, it is necessary to study patients with simpler and milder disorders than most patients encountered in clinical practice who will actually receive the drug (Bodenheimer, 2000). Samples in industry-sponsored research are homogeneous groups who score above a minimum symptom rating scale score and who do not have complicating features such as comorbidity, which limits generalizability of the findings (Zimmerman, Chelminski, & Posternak, 2004). For example, just 4–8% of Alzheimer's disease patients in clinical settings met criteria for two large clinical trials of drugs for this condition (Lagomasino et al., 2005). Phase III studies of major depression exclude patients with chronicity, comorbidity, suicide risk, psychosis, or bipolar illness. Bipolar studies usually enroll patients with remitted mania or bipolar I depression, not rapid or ultradian cycling or chronic symptoms; in fact, how many seriously ill bipolar patients would be able to maintain consent to remain in a study for any length of time? The fact that all of these studies exclude patients with active substance use means that 50–70% of patients usually seen in clinical practice are not studied.

"Sample enrichment," or selecting a subpopulation that is more likely to demonstrate effectiveness of the study medication, is a good strategy when it is used to test the hypothesis that a treatment will only work for a particular subtype. This strategy was very enlightening in a study of gefitinib, an experimental anticancer drug (Lynch, 2004). Gefitinib is an antagonist of a receptor for epidermal growth factor (EGF), which stimulates growth of cancer cells. While this very expensive and toxic drug did not work for most patients with chemotherapy-resistant non–small cell lung cancer, 10–19% of patients seemed to be cured by it. The investigators found that of the 9 of 275 patients in clinical trials who did have an excellent response to gefitinib, 8 had over-lapping heterozygous mutations in the tyrosine kinase domain of the EGF receptor, which happens to be the same site to which gefitinib binds. As it turned out, these mutations made the EGF receptor 10 times as sensitive to gefitinib, which would theoreti-cally make the drug more effective in blocking the receptor and inhibiting tumor growth; the same mutations could increase sen-sitivity of the receptor to EGF and make lung tumors grow faster.

With this information, the investigators designed a prospec-tive blinded study of the drug in patients with treatment-resistant lung cancer who had the EGF receptor gene muta-tion. The drug worked in the majority of this subgroup. Now, lung cancer patients who have not responded to the usual treat-ments can be genotyped for the EGF receptor gene. If they have the mutation that predicts a response to gefitinib, they can be given the drug. Otherwise, they are spared the expense and side effects of a medication that is highly unlikely to produce any benefit.

Choosing specific subtypes for a prospective study, for exam-ple, patients with bipolar mood disorders, would be a very useful strategy for identifying markers of a preferential response (or lack of it) to one treatment or another. However, most industry sponsored psychopharmacology studies do not use sample en-richment for this purpose. Instead, they try to pick patients who are most likely to respond to the study drug by eliminating everyone who does not do well on the treatment in an open trial, whereas those who seem to respond go on to a double-blind study. For example, manic patients with an initial response to a particular antipsychotic drug in open treatment might then be randomized to take that medication or a placebo, while patients who did not do well acutely do not go into the double-blind study. The only valid conclusion from this kind of study is that patients who respond at first may be more likely to respond again, not that the treatment is more likely than a placebo to work in any patient who walks in the door.

CAN WE GENERALIZE FROM
INDUSTRY-SPONSORED TRIALS
TO OUR PATIENTS?

Along with selection of patients with uncomplicated illnesses, sample enrichment, and lack of complete correction for dropouts, recent studies of new treatments are plagued by a shortage of subjects with significant cases of the target condition. As more therapies have become available for psychiatric disorders, patients with simpler disorders have had a wider choice of effective therapies, and they are understandably more reluctant to enroll in a study in which they might get a placebo. To meet enrollment criteria, centers now recruit subjects via advertisements, many of whom are "symptomatic volunteers." Symptomatic volunteers have actual symptoms, but they are not particularly ill and therefore they are not necessarily comparable with clinical populations who seek treatment (Zimmerman et al., 2004). The need to recruit such subjects is increased when companies offer bonuses for reaching enrollment targets for clinical trials, increasing the recruitment of subjects who technically meet entry criteria but are not as ill as patients in clinical practice (Angell, 2005). How do all of these factors affect the applicability to our patients of the results of the studies we frequently read?

A review of 39 antidepressant efficacy studies published from 1994 to 2000 in five prominent journals applied the exclusion criteria used in the studies to a sample of 596 depressed patients seeking outpatient treatment in a university clinic (Zimmerman et al., 2004). Because these patients were enrolled in another study, they received structured diagnostic interviews, HDRSs, and personality disorder interviews, so a good deal of information about them was available. Exclusion criteria in the efficacy studies included HDRS score below a certain level, suicide risk, psychotic features or history of psychosis, substance abuse, bipolar disorder, dysthymic disorder, short (1 month) or long (1–2 years) depressive episodes, borderline personality disorder, and comorbid Axis I disorder. Applying all of these exclusion criteria to their sample, the authors found that 9.9% would be excluded because of bipolar disorder, 5.7% for psychotic features, 47% for HDRS score below

20, 8.9% for substance use disorder in the previous 6 months, 6.6% for suicidality, 55.5% for comorbid anxiety disorder, 10% for borderline personality disorder, 9% for dysthymic disorder, and 8% for another Axis I disorder; episode duration was 2–3 weeks in 6.4%, 43.9% had an episode that had lasted more than 12 months, and 32% had an episode lasting more than 2 years. Overall, an average of 65.8% of the clinic patients would have been excluded from the reported clinical trials. More than 90% of the clinic patients would have been excluded from two of the published studies. The actual number of patients excluded from the published trials may have been even higher since many studies use unreported exclusion criteria such as comorbid medical illness, engagement in psychotherapy, or lack of adequate contraception. In addition, while most industry-sponsored studies report how many patients drop out, they do not report how many patients were screened in order to get an adequate sample. This is a very important detail because it tells us how much the deck was stacked in favor of the study drug by enriching the sample and what percent of the actual clinical population is represented by the subjects.

Even if subjects have clinically relevant illnesses, the primary outcome measures in Phase III clinical trials may not be entirely relevant clinically. The goal of most of these studies is to demonstrate a statistically significant reduction of scores on a symptom rating scale such as the HDRS or the PANSS, perhaps with the additional aim of demonstrating that more patients had a sufficient reduction to qualify for response or remission. The premise that being 50% less symptomatic is a desirable goal or that reduction of symptoms is an indication that the patient is really well has no empirical basis and in fact is contradicted by research, which indicates that inadequate functional outcome predicts later relapse of the full syndrome. Even if it were true that symptom reduction is illness cure, the question arises whether the rating scales actually measure symptomatic outcome adequately. The HDRS, which contains multiple items related to anxiety and insomnia and just one on suicidality, is one of the mainstays of antidepressant clinical trials. Yet in a careful criticism of the validity and reliability of the HDRS, Bagby, Michael,

Ryder, Schuller, & Marshall commented on "the marked contrast between the effort and scientific sophistication involved in designing new antidepressants and the continued reliance on antiquated concepts and methods for assessing change in the severity of the depression that these very medications are intended to affect (2004, pp. 2174–2175).

Just as it is important to evaluate the clinical relevance of the sample in clinical trials, it is necessary to evaluate the clinical relevance of doses of reference medications in studies that demonstrate equivalence with newer medications. Not infrequently, the comparison standard is underdosed (Bodenheimer, 2000). Most studies of atypical antipsychotic drugs that compare them to haloperidol or occasionally to clozapine, for instance, do not adjust doses of the older medications by blood level although both are thought to have correlations between blood level and clinical response. Comparisons of new mood stabilizers to lithium often use lower lithium levels than would be used in clinical practice.

To provide clinically relevant evidence, randomized trials should recruit heterogeneous groups of patients in which there is substantial clinical uncertainty about the best treatment for a particular patient, randomized trials must also be large enough to detect moderately sized treatment effects, and they must measure outcomes of clear clinical importance (Geddes & Goodwin, 2001). However, most trials in psychiatry are performed for regulatory purposes on relatively homogeneous samples, which requires a smaller number of patients than studies designed to detect important clinical effects in the larger population of patients (Geddes & Goodwin, 2001). For example, considering reported recurrence rates and dropout rates and assuming that a 10% difference between treatments is clinically meaningful, a reasonably powered study comparing lithium and valproate would have 2,100 to 3,000 patients (Geddes & Goodwin, 2001). In contrast, most clinical trials in psychiatry enroll at most a few hundred patients; the CATIE study (see pp. 56–57) was remarkable in enrolling approximately 1,400 patients.

ARE THE RESULTS OF INDUSTRY-SPONSORED TRIALS BIASED?

The majority (89–98%) of published industry-sponsored medication comparisons favor the sponsor's product (Carpenter, 2002; Montgomery et al., 2004). A review conducted in 2002 of 72 industry-sponsored and 14 non-industry-sponsored RCTs comparing second-generation ("atypical") antipsychotic drugs to other medications (Montgomery et al., 2004) found that even though the quality of design was equally good in industry-sponsored and non-industry-sponsored trials, the non-industry-sponsored trials were significantly more likely to include equivalence of the industry product and the comparison drug in the 95% CI. In other words, the industry-sponsored studies found that their product was at least as good as existing products while the independent studies did not. Of the trials that were reviewed, 70% compared atypicals to the older neuroleptics such as haloperidol, and 13 trials were head-to-head comparisons of atypicals; however, 8 of the latter were "non-inferiority" comparisons with clozapine that were designed to show that the new drug was not worse than clozapine and therefore did not restrict the sample to patients with truly refractory illnesses. Comparisons to clozapine that were not funded by industry were much more likely than industry-sponsored studies to include seriously treatment-resistant patients. The industry-sponsored studies therefore may have been designed to show that their products were not worse than clozapine in any patient, whereas the independent studies seem to have been more likely to have been designed to examine efficacy in more severely ill patients, in which case clozapine performed better.

Although some research suggests that industry-sponsored trials are of lower quality, and low-quality trials overestimate therapeutic benefit by an average of 34% (Djulbegovic et al., 2000), many reviews find that quality of research is not the explanation for the tendency of industry-sponsored clinical trials to find that their products are better than reference medications or the newer competition. In a study of 159 RCTs published in the *BMJ* from 1997 to 2001, studies funded by for-profit companies were significantly more likely to favor the experimental treatment, compared with trials with no industry support, nonprofit support, or combinations of for-profit and nonprofit support (Kjaergard & Als-Nielsen, 2002). The difference was not explained by authors' affiliations, methodological quality, statistical power, specialty, or type of intervention and control.

A similar study examined 332 randomized trials published between 1999 and 2001 in eight leading surgical journals and five leading medical journals (Bhandari et al., 2004). Industry-funded trials were 1.9 times as likely as other studies to have findings favoring the new industry product, an increase that remained significant when corrected for study quality and sample size. Medical and surgical trials were equally likely to have this kind of pro-industry result (Bhandari et al., 2004).

A review of 397 controlled trials published over a 2-year period in four widely cited psychiatric journals found that 60% of studies reported at least some industry support, 18% reported other private support, 25% reported public support, and 19% reported no support; many studies reported multiple funding sources (Perlis et al., 2005). Industry support itself was not associated with results favoring the company's drug, but if the author had any conflict of interest (even consulting to the company), it was five to eight times as likely that positive findings about a new drug would be reported. In contrast, there was no association between author conflict of interest and results in non-industry-supported studies.

To get a better picture of the influence of industry sponsorship by not bundling different kinds of studies, studies were reviewed of treatment of a single illness in which a good deal of research has occurred—multiple myeloma (Djulbegovic et al., 2000). After looking for all randomized trials for multiple myeloma between 1996 and 1998, 113 articles describing 136 trials were found. The authors hypothesized that if there was true uncertainty about the benefit of new treatments, the latter should be found to be more effective than the comparison treatment about as frequently as they were found not to be more effective, considering both benefit and harm. Almost three fourths (72%) of the trials were of poor quality, and only 5% were of high quality. Overall, equal numbers of studies favored new therapies and standard therapies. However, when trials were analyzed according to support by commercial versus nonprofit organizations, 74% of studies with commercial support favored the new product versus 53% of studies with nonprofit support. In addition, more industry-sponsored studies compared a new treatment to a placebo or no therapy than did studies with federal support (60% versus 21%), and the experimental treatment was favored in 70–90% of studies in which the comparator was a placebo. This finding was not a function of industry-sponsored studies being of lower quality, since they were as good as non-industry-sponsored studies; it was just that the studies were designed to favor the new drug. And why wouldn't industry be more likely to fund studies with a greater chance of finding superiority of their product?

There are a number of additional reasons for the tendency of industry-sponsored trials to find that their products are superior (Montgomery et al., 2004). We have already discussed the use of a dose of a comparison drug that is not really comparable to the dose of the study drug. Another possibility is that when negative results begin to emerge, the study is discontinued, or perhaps negative results are not submitted for publication.

The process of publication of results of large multicenter industry-sponsored studies can add to their tendency to present a less than neutral view of the product that was tested. As we saw on page 68, the principal investigator in a large clinical trial in which a manufacturer, often through a CRO, subcontracts with sites around the world to enroll patients, either works for the company or has a relationship with it that is sufficiently extensive for the company to have confidence that they share the same view of the research being conducted. There is nothing nefarious about this—any rational group would want to do business with someone it knows and trusts, but the arrangement does result in one or perhaps a small number of investigators having access to all of the data. The large number of investigators who carry out the study usually do not see any of the results. In fact, they never find out which of their patients got which treatment unless there is an emergency and the blind has to be broken. Even when raw data are made available to the investigators, the initial tabulation of data is performed by the company or a CRO, often in a manner that can skew the data interpretation (Healy & Cattell, 2003).

The small group that reviews all the data with company oversight decides what to publish and writes up the results. Once a research report is drafted, the other investigators may have a chance to comment on it, but even if their comments were integrated into the article it would be impossible for them to critique the report intelligently since they have not seen the entire body of data, including the unpublished data. The informed reader of such reports—in other words, of most reports of industry-sponsored Phase III and Phase IV trials—should be aware of two outcomes of this process.

One phenomenon that occurs frequently when a large clinical trial is completed involves multiple publications of the same study, often with rotating authorship (Montgomery et al., 2004). When practitioners see a number of articles with different lead authors that all describe about the same result, they may conclude that independent groups have all found that a new product is better than its comparators. This impression is even more deceptive when each of a number of articles reports part of the data from the same large trial, each one presenting a slightly different facet of the findings. A meta-analysis then includes more than one version of the same study, inflating estimates of a new drug's benefit (Montgomery et al., 2004).

The second outcome of closed review of data is the decision not to publish negative results, which may include lack of efficacy in important domains, adverse effects, or the entire study. Publication bias, or the selective publication of positive results, has been found not to result from journals not wanting to publish negative results, but from authors deciding not to submit them (Montgomery et al., 2004).

Selective publication played an important role in the widespread acceptance of the cyclooxygenase-2 (COX-2) inhibitors as having a lower risk of gastrointestinal (GI) bleeding than the first-generation nonsteroidal anti-inflammatory drugs such as ibuprofen. Manufacturer-sponsored investigators published data from the first 6 months of a large multicenter study that indicated a lower risk of GI bleeding with Celebrex than with ibuprofen, but the full study, which lasted 12 months and found no difference in GI side effects between the drugs, was not published (Abramson, 2004). Similarly, a large study that compared Vioxx with naproxen, published its finding of significantly fewer serious adverse GI effects with the new medication but did not publish the finding of significantly more adverse cardiovascular complications (Abramson, 2004). The rigorous peer review of the prestigious medical journals that published these studies did not detect the lack of completeness of the data.

One estimate is that 11% of reports of industry-sponsored multicenter trials in peer-reviewed journals are not just written by investigators who work for the company, but are ghostwritten by industry personnel (Healy & Cattell, 2003), and 19% of reports have authors who did not contribute materially to the study (Bodenheimer, 2000). Such articles name as an author an investigator who never analyzed—and may not even have seen— the data but they do not list the ghostwriter (Bodenheimer, 2000). In some cases, a well-known guest author has final say over the publication but does not necessarily review it carefully (Bodenheimer, 2000). A study of this question found that authors of published industry-sponsored studies of sertraline had more of an impact on readers and were published in more prestigious journals than sertraline studies that did not seem to have such support (Healy & Cattell, 2003). This may simply mean that industry-sponsored studies utilize more capable and prominent researchers, but in the case of sertraline, the combination of prestigious journals, prestigious authors, more widespread distribution (by industry representatives) of the industry-sponsored articles, and sponsored symposia summarizing the studies had 50% more impact on the field than the nonsponsored articles of sertraline. At the same time, selective publication was manifested by the 9% of patients in pediatric studies who had increased suicidality being omitted from the publications of those studies (Healy & Cattell, 2003).

4

How to Interpret
Research Studies

One reason why it is important to understand how industry-sponsored studies and the articles that report their results are designed is that industry is heavily involved in much of the research we rely on to guide prescribing. Of course, research that is not funded by industry may have similar design issues. Design issues in influential studies do not invalidate them, but a knowledge of research design allows us to place them in proper perspective in our clinical decision making.

Using research in clinical practice involves precisely defining a patient problem, deciding what information is needed to resolve the problem, conducting an efficient literature search, selecting the best of the relevant studies, applying rules of evidence to determine the validity of studies that are reviewed, being able to extract the clinical message, and applying this to the patient problem (Group, 1992). When reading studies of a new treatment (or when hearing about them in a 5-minute presentation by an industry representative), these questions can help to decide how much confidence to have in treatment (Dans, Dans, Guyatt, & Richardson, 1998; Guyatt et al., 1994):

- Are the results of the study likely to be valid? That is, do the results represent an unbiased estimate of the treatment effect, or is there a systematic influence toward a false conclusion? The answer to this question depends on:
  ○ Randomly assigning patients to the treatment conditions. Any other method is more likely to show larger and false positive treatment effects. If there are no randomized trials for a specific therapeutic question, the clinician has to

rely on weaker studies. This is usually the case for new treatments or new applications of a treatment. For example, gabapentin (Neurontin) was first suggested as a treatment for bipolar disorder based on a few case series, and many clinicians adopted it. Industry representatives could not promote the product for this indication without FDA approval, but they could provide copies of the articles supporting its use. Then controlled studies showed that it did not work, and clinical experience demonstrated that it sometimes made patients more manic, but this has not stopped some clinicians from continuing to use it as a mood stabilizer.

○ Properly accounting for all patients at the end of the study. Several steps must be taken to ensure complete data collection, and it is important that none of these steps is skipped.

- Performing a complete follow-up. If substantial numbers of patients are lost to follow-up, the validity of the study is questionable, because patients who leave the study may be different from those who remain, and it is not known whether they dropped out because of adverse outcomes or because they were well. The safest assumption is that in positive trials, all patients lost from the treatment group did badly and all lost from the control group did well. If recalculating the outcomes under these assumptions does not change the conclusions, the loss to follow-up was not a problem. If it is too much trouble to do this calculation, ask the representative to get the information. Simply stating that dropouts did not differ from patients who remained in the study in their baseline characteristics is not sufficiently reassuring to omit this recalculation.

- Including all randomized patients in the analysis. It is important to include noncompliant patients in the data analysis because these patients have been found to have a worse prognosis, even when all relevant risk factors are controlled and the treatment is a placebo. Data from these patients must be included in both

groups—just including noncompliant patients in the
control group will make the experimental treatment
seem better than is really the case.

- Adequately blinding patients, clinicians, and study personnel. In some studies, it is impossible to blind patients
  and clinicians. In these cases, the raters should at least be
  blinded.

- Ensuring that the groups were similar at the start of the
  trial.

- Treating all groups in the same manner. This is especially
  difficult when a new treatment is added to "treatment as
  usual," which often differs from patient to patient.

- How large was the treatment effect? As a general rule, the
  larger the sample size, the greater the confidence that the
  true measure of efficacy is close to the observed efficacy
  measure; in other words, that the 95% CI contains the result of this study. The narrower the 95% CI around the result, the more confidence one can have in the result. Another point to bear in mind is that if the lower end of the
  95% CI is clinically important (i.e., that even if the lowest
  estimate of efficacy would make a difference in treatment),
  the sample size was large enough. If not, the study is not
  definitive, even if the results are statistically significant. For
  example, if the active drug was twice as effective as placebo
  and the 95% CI is 1.1–3, the lowest estimate is that the active drug was just a little better than placebo and the result
  must be taken with a large grain of salt. Similarly, if the upper boundary of the 95% CI of a negative study would be
  clinically important if it were the real result, the study has
  not excluded the possibility of an important treatment effect that was missed.

- Will the results help me to take care of my patients? The answer to this question depends on the similarity of your patients to the patients in the study, and whether the outcome
  is important to them. It is necessary to balance benefits and
  risks of the treatment and the consequences of withholding
  treatment. An effective therapy might be withheld if the patients' prognosis is good without treatment and if the treat-

ment has the potential for significant toxicity. To address whether the potential benefit actually applies to your patients, first decide whether your patients resemble the ones in the study by determining whether your patients meet all of the inclusion criteria and none of the exclusion criteria in a study. If your patients are a little outside the study criteria— for example, if they were a few years too old or too young or had previously been treated with a competing therapy—the study results are still likely to be relevant. Additional considerations in determining whether the study does not apply to one's patients include:

○ If the treatment did not work in the overall sample but the investigators retrospectively examined subgroups in an attempt to prove that the treatment works for a particular group (subgroup analysis), it is easier to believe that similar patients in your practice might also respond if:

- There was a large difference in treatment effect between subgroups.
- The difference is very unlikely to have occurred by chance.
- There was a hypothesis before the study began that the subgroup would respond preferentially.
- A small number of subgroup analyses were carried out.
- The subgroup difference is replicated in other studies.

○ There may be important differences between the illness the clinician is treating and the illness in the study. For example, most RCTs of acute treatment of bipolar disorder involve 3-week trials in mania comparing a new medication (e.g., an atypical antipsychotic drug) with a placebo, and sometimes also with an active comparator such as divalproex. Such studies would not necessarily apply to hypomanic patients, or to manic patients who would not be competent or willing to enroll in a placebo controlled study. Since many manic patients refuse to take medication in the first place or even to stay in the hospital voluntarily, many seriously manic patients would not qualify for a RCT. Similarly, maintenance studies usually involve patients with bipolar I disorder who are stable at the time of randomization and who do well acutely to an open trial of the new medication, when more patients in clinical practice have bipolar II disorder, are ill at the time treatment is begun, and have difficulty responding to a single treatment. Even within a specific categorical diagnosis, there is a broad spectrum of disorders with different treatment responses. Bipolar disorder with frequent recurrences and unstable interepisode functioning that started in childhood may respond to different treatments than later-onset bipolar disorder with few episodes and good baseline functioning.

○ Most large RCTs in psychiatry systematically exclude patients with comorbid conditions who are likely to have entirely different treatment responses. For example, a comorbid substance use disorder can drastically reduce the response to any treatment if it is not addressed at the same time. In addition, because they are followed more closely and their compliance is repeatedly assessed (not to mention that they are willing to participate in a study in the first place), adherence to a treatment protocol by subjects in a study is usually greater than it is in patients in office practice. Practical factors (e.g., not being able to afford the medication) and psychological factors (e.g., not wanting to rely on the doctor's treatment) result in at least half of patients in real-life practice not taking medications as prescribed (Keck, McElroy, Strakowski, Bourne, & West, 1997; Melfi et al., 1998).

○ Patients from ethnic or social groups different from the study population may have higher or lower baseline rates of illness or may be more or less likely to improve spontaneously, altering the relative risk reduction and therefore the NNT in our patients.

○ Pharmacokinetic and pharmacodynamic factors are usually not studied in RCTs, but knowledge is accumulating that there is a wide distribution of activity of genes that influence drug metabolism and drug effect in the general population. Until more information becomes available, we will not be able to be certain about how likely our patients will be able to metabolize the medication in a manner similar to the patients in the study.

○ Perhaps the most important factor in assessing the usefulness to our patients of a new study is whether clinically important outcomes were considered. Physiological or rating scale measures are often used as substitute endpoints for clinically important measures such as functioning because confirming benefit on the latter would require more patients followed for a longer period of time with more detailed observation. However, the substitute endpoint might not really reflect the clinically desirable one. Also, improvement in one important outcome may be balanced by deleterious effects on other outcomes. A dramatic example of this kind of problem occurred in the CASTs. The Type Ia antiarrhythmic drugs (e.g., quinidine, procainamide, and disopyramide suppressed the substitute endpoint of abnormal ventricular depolarizations in randomized trials, but in studies of whether this translated into fewer arrhythmias after M.I., it turned out that these medications *increased* the mortality rate. In contrast, beta-blockers did reduce the risk of sudden death. This particular study has some relevance for psychiatry since the tricyclic antidepressants are also Type Ia antiarrhythmics.

- Are there important differences from the study in provider compliance? Like patients, clinicians are usually more motivated to ensure and follow treatment adherence when they are involved in a clinical trial than they are in everyday practice. A clinician may not be familiar or comfortable with the treatment used in the study and is likely to be less motivated than an investigator to encourage patients to continue a treatment that is causing side effects. Busy clinicians may be less likely to call patients who miss an appointment to be sure they come right in than are investigators who need patients to complete a study.
- Are the likely benefits of treatment worth the potential harms and costs? The lower the NNT, the greater the likely benefit. The NNT for benefit must be balanced against the

number needed to harm (NNH). For example, if a beta-blocker causes clinically important fatigue in 10% (0.1) of patients, the NNT for fatigue is $1/0.1 = 10$. If a beta-blocker has a NNT of 400 per life saved as a result of reducing the risk of arrhythmia after M.I., 40 patients will be fatigued for every life that is saved. In low-risk patients who have not had a recent M.I., 400 would be fatigued to save one life. The risk of discontinuing the drug in fatigued patients at low risk of cardiovascular death would therefore be less than in patients with a higher baseline mortality risk. In psychiatric studies, we have little information about the balance between the number of adverse events per positive outcome based on the likelihood that the treatment will help the patient, so this decision often involves a good deal of guesswork.

II
Practice

5

Analyzing Studies That Influence Treatment Choice

This chapter demonstrates how the principles we have been reviewing can be used to understand what to make of the research we come across every day by applying them to a few of the more influential studies that have been published recently, and the interpretation of these studies for marketing purposes. The same principles apply to industry-sponsored and non-industry-sponsored studies.

SCHIZOPHRENIA

The atypical antipsychotics rapidly captured a large market share, despite being 10 times more expensive than the neuroleptics, because they were reported to be better tolerated, superior for negative symptoms, and useful for treatment resistance (Carpenter, 2002). However, the FDA never approved any claim for superior efficacy in refractory schizophrenia of any atypical antipsychotic except clozapine, and federally supported studies do not support greater efficacy of the newer atypical antipsychotics for negative symptoms. Some experts feel that any apparent superiority of the newer drugs may be the result of the new products producing fewer negative effects than haloperidol, the standard comparison drug, in registration trials (Carpenter, 2002). In most of these studies, haloperidol is given in doses that are high enough to produce akinesia and affective blunting, which can be very difficult to distinguish from negative symptoms. Haloperidol has been found to have a relationship between blood level and clinical response, but blood levels are virtually never used when a new antipsychotic drug is compared with haloperidol.

It turns out that not all studies show that patients like the atypical antipsychotic drugs better when careful dosing of the older drugs is used. In these situations, dropout rates are often similar for atypical antipsychotics and the older drugs. The atypical may improve cognition, but this finding could simply be the result of producing less "cognitive parkinsonism" than haloperidol as the comparison drug (Carpenter, 2002). These impressions were supported by a collaborative study at 17 VA medical centers in a real-life clinical setting following a study algorithm that found no significant differences between olanzapine and haloperidol plus benztropine in study retention, positive, negative, or total symptoms, or quality of life; olanzapine was less likely to cause extrapyramidal side effects but more likely to cause weight gain, and it cost significantly more (Rosenheck, Davis, Evans, & Herz, 2003). So far, the risk of tardive dyskinesia does appear to be lower with the atypical antipsychotics, but tardive dyskinesia only became apparent with the neuroleptics after decades of use, and the newer drugs may have more metabolic and possibly cerebrovascular risks. Based on clinical experience, the atypicals are still appropriate first-line treatments for schizophrenia, but understanding antipsychotic drug studies makes it apparent that the last word is far from in.

In one of the first federally funded studies of the real-world use of antipsychotic drugs (Lieberman et al., 2005)—the CATIE trial—1,493 chronic schizophrenia patients (of whom data were available for 1,432) were randomly assigned to take the older neuroleptic perphenazine (mean dose 21 mg/day) or the new antipsychotic drugs olanzapine (mean dose 20 mg/day), risperidone (mean dose 4 mg/day), quetiapine (mean dose 543 mg/day), or, later in the study when it was approved by the FDA, ziprasidone (mean dose 113 mg/day); aripiprazole had not yet been released at the time of the study. Doses were adjusted according to side effects and response. The primary outcome measure was time to discontinuation of treatment, which was felt to be a real-life indicator of how patients do in practice since if they do not take a medication, it is not likely to work. The authors also looked at symptom rating scales, side effects, and a variety of other secondary outcomes.

A total of 74% of the patients discontinued their medication for any reason before the 18 months of the study were over, ranging from 64% discontinuing olanzapine to 82% discontinuing quetiapine. It appeared that the time to medication discontinuation was statistically significantly longer for olanzapine than the other medications (i.e., that patients stayed on olanzapine longer), but when corrections were made for the multiple statistical tests that were done, it turned out that there was no difference between olanzapine and perphenazine in time to treatment discontinuation. It also seemed at first that patients were more likely to stay on olanzapine than ziprasidone, but this difference was not significant either when the appropriate adjustments for multiple comparisons were made in the statistical analysis. Patients were less likely to discontinue olanzapine than medications other than ziprasidone, but the absolute differences were not great: 15% discontinued olanzapine for lack of efficacy versus 28% quetiapine, 27% risperidone, 25% perphenazine, and 24% ziprasidone. These percentage differences might seem great until one realizes that the absolute numbers in each group were not substantial and there were no differences in likelihood of medication discontinuation because of patient preference or side effects, including the extrapyramidal side effects that are generally considered to be much less of a problem with the atypicals. At the same time, significantly more patients taking olanzapine gained more than 7% of their baseline weight (considered clinically important weight gain) than the other medications (30% of olanzapine patients versus 10–15% of patients taking the other medications), and patients gained an average of 9.4 pounds on olanzapine versus 1.1 pounds weight gain to 2.0 pounds weight loss with the other antipsychotic drugs; cholesterol and triglyceride levels also increased significantly more with olanzapine.

In industry-sponsored talks, the manufacturer of olanzapine has been touting its product's superiority over other antipsychotic drugs because the CATIE trial showed that patients stayed on olanzapine longer, leading to lower symptom rating scale scores of unclear clinical importance. It might be worth bearing in mind in interpreting this claim that the average dose of olanzapine was proportionately higher than that of the other medications. And when more than two thirds of patients cannot stay on your medication for 18 months it is hardly something to brag about, especially when patients who stay on the medication gain significant amounts of weight and develop evidence of metabolic abnormalities. The real take-home messages of the CATIE study is that (a) most schizophrenia patients do not continue any medications that have been proven in controlled studies to help their symptoms, and (b) the superiority of the atypical antipsychotics that appears in promotional material is far from dramatic.

The British Cost Utility of the Latest Antipsychotic Drugs in Schizophrenia Study (CUTLASS I) supported the impression suggested by CATIE that industry-sponsored Phase III and Phase IV studies do not replicate the conditions in which practitioners actually work and do not necessarily measure outcomes that reflect how patients are actually doing (Jones et al., 2006). This study randomized 227 chronic schizophrenia patients to a neuroleptic or first-generation antipsychotic drug (FGA) or an atypical second-generation antipsychotic drug (SGA) for one year. Medications and doses were chosen by patients' psychiatrists, and if a switch was necessary, every attempt was made to change to a new medication in the same class. The primary outcome measure was a well validated, blindly rated quality of life scale that assessed multiple aspects of social, psychological, and occupational functioning; secondary measures included symptoms and side effects. Since 81% of the patients could be assessed at the end of the study, the dropout rate was lower than in the CATIE trial.

After a year of treatment, there was no significant difference in quality of life scores between FGAs and SGAs. Even more startling, there were no significant differences between drug classes in extrapyramidal side effects, compliance, attitudes toward medication, PANSS scores (including negative symptom subscales), depression, or global assessment of functioning. The total cost of care was statistically equivalent for both groups, with the actual cost of medication being only 2% of the total cost of care for FGAs and 4% for SGAs. Had marketing of the newer medications been less intense, perhaps the dismay clinicians felt at this result would have been less marked.

BIPOLAR DISORDER

The anticonvulsant lamotrigine has gained popularity as a treatment for bipolar disorder based on several multicenter, industry-sponsored, controlled trials. In a 7-week double-blind study of 195 patients with bipolar I depression, both 50 and 200 mg/day of lamotrigine were equivalently superior to placebo in reducing Montgomery-Asberg Depression Rating Scale (MADRS) scores when observed cases were considered, but only 200 mg was superior to placebo in an intent-to-treat (LOCF) model (Calabrese et al., 1999). About half of the patients on lamotrigine versus one fourth on placebo had a response, and average MADRS scores decreased by about 50%; remission rates, other symptoms, and actual functioning were not provided. In a 52-week continuation of this study, all patients were treated openly with lamotrigine, usually as an adjunct along with other medications deemed necessary by the treating physician (McElroy et al., 2004). Improvement of depression appeared to be sustained without mood destabilization. This seemed like a good start to studies of a medication that might not be as likely as standard antidepressants to make bipolar mood disorders worse.

In one of the two pivotal (i.e., used for regulatory approval) industry-sponsored lamotrigine trials in bipolar depression (Bowden et al., 2003), 349 recently manic or hypomanic but currently improved bipolar I patients were switched over 6 weeks from whatever treatment they were receiving to lamotrigine for an 8-to-16-week open-label phase. Half of the sample (175 patients) continued to do well on lamotrigine and this group was then randomized for 18 months to lamotrigine (50, 200, or 400 mg/day), lithium (serum level 0.8–1.1 mM), or placebo; the half that did not do well with open-label lamotrigine was dropped from the study. For the patients who continued on lamotrigine, the 50-mg dose was ineffective, but the two higher doses were both significantly more likely than placebo to lengthen the time to recurrence of depressive symptoms without any increase in manic symptoms: over the 18 months, 36% of lamotrigine patients versus 27% of placebo patients did not require an additional intervention for depression. In contrast, lithium but not lamotrigine was significantly better than placebo in lengthening the time to a new intervention for a manic episode, without any increase in the risk of recurrence of depression. The generalizability of this finding is limited by the use of sample enrichment, which excluded half the initial sample and only enrolled patients in the double-blind phase who did well with open treatment with lamotrigine. Furthermore, patients were not acutely ill at the onset of the double-blind phase, and only bipolar I depression was studied. The most generous conclusion is that half of a group of bipolar I patients who are willing to stay in a study for 18 months and who are already doing well on any treatment—in other words, a fairly stable population— can stay on lamotrigine for up to 4 months, and that staying on lamotrigine is associated with 9% more lamotrigine than placebo patients not needing more treatment for depression during that time.

A similar methodology was used in the other lamotrigine pivotal trial. In this study, currently or recently depressed bipolar I outpatients were treated openly with lamotrigine titrated up to 200 mg/day while other medications were withdrawn (Calabrese et al., 2003). Of 966 patients enrolled in the study, less than half (463) survived (i.e., stayed in) the open-label phase. These patients were then randomly assigned to 50, 200, or 400 mg/day of lamotrigine, lithium (0.8–1.1 mM), or placebo for 18 months. Lamotrigine and lithium both prolonged the time to intervention of any mood episode significantly more than placebo, with the active treatments appearing equivalently effective for this purpose.

When data from the two latter studies were combined (Goodwin et al., 2004), lamotrigine suddenly appeared to be significantly more likely than placebo to lengthen the time to intervention for a new manic episode even though this was not the case in either study alone, leading to FDA approval as a maintenance treatment for bipolar disorder. If retrospective combination of two studies with negative findings and different patient populations (recently manic/hypomanic versus recently depressed) to produce a positive finding were to be performed for any other illness, it would be considered far from compelling. Apparently, the standard of proof for a psychiatric illness is not as high. It is also worth noting that the time to an affective recurrence in either direction on lamotrigine was 197 days, indicating that the average lamotrigine-treated patient went 6 months before having a recurrence—hardly a finding to revolutionize treatment even if the statistical analysis were valid and clinically relevant. Since the large controlled trials only considered patients with bipolar I mood disorders who are very unlikely to have had malignant or complex courses given their ability to enroll and remain in the study, more information is necessary before clinicians can be confident that this medication is really a mood stabilizer for the average complex patient in clinical practice.

A study sponsored by the manufacturer and conducted by a number of investigators some of whom were employees of or stockholders in the company examined whether adding olanzapine to lithium or valproate in patients who had already responded to the mood stabilizer would help to reduce the risk of a recurrence (Tohen et al., 2004). This study involved 344 patients with pure or mixed mania who had been treated in another study for an average of 67 days with therapeutic levels of lithium or valproate combined with olanzapine or placebo. About half (160) of these patients had been given lithium or valproate plus olanzapine. Of the group that had received olanzapine plus one of the standard mood stabilizers, 61 were excluded, 58 of them because they did not achieve a remission. The remaining 99 patients who met the authors' definition of remission (manic symptoms that were significantly less severe) after having received olanzapine plus one of the mood stabilizers were rerandomized to take lithium or valproate plus olanzapine (51 patients) or a placebo for the next 18 months.

Only 16 of the patients who took olanzapine plus a mood stabilizer completed the study, while more than two thirds (35) withdrew. This result was not substantially better than the result with those who took a mood stabilizer plus a placebo: 43 of the latter 48 patients withdrew from the study and 10% (5 patients) completed it. The median time to dropping out of the study was 111 days with olanzapine add-on and 82 days with placebo add-on. The same percentage in each group withdrew because of lack of efficacy. There was also no difference between groups in time to syndromic relapse or in the rate of syndromic relapse into mania or depression. Looking for something that might be statistically significant, the researchers found that the median time to symptomatic relapse was 163 days for olanzapine add-on versus 42 days for placebo add-on, a difference that was explained entirely by results in female and Caucasian patients. While the time to relapse was longer with olanzapine add-on, there was no difference between olanzapine and placebo add-on groups in the *rate* of symptomatic relapse. The report emphasized the benefit of adding olanzapine in lengthening the time it took for an affective relapse to occur.

The protocols for evaluating clinical trials that we have been reviewing make the weaknesses of this study apparent. For one thing, the study was enriched by eliminating almost 40% of acutely treated olanzapine patients. Any conclusion that could be drawn would not apply to all patients receiving addition of olanzapine for mood stabilization, but only those who are able to stay on the medication for the first couple of months. We are not provided with enough details about the patients who were studied to know how well they resemble the patients we treat, but it is a reasonable bet that not all of our patients would be willing to enroll in an 18-month study. Indeed, many have difficulty making an ongoing commitment to treatment, and those who do often take more than one mood stabilizer in the first place. Most remarkable, however, is that the initial assumption about the number of dropouts, which was essential to the power analysis that determined how many patients it would be necessary to enroll to obtain a significant result, was wrong. Having acknowledged this fact, the investigators went on to present their results as though the initial statistical assumption was correct.

What were those results? Almost 70% of patients did not stay on olanzapine, mainly because adding it was not effective. The primary outcome measure—rate of relapse into mania, depression, or any affective episode—was no better with olanzapine than with placebo add-on. Patients taking olanzapine plus lithium or valproate remained in the study 29 days longer than those having placebo added, but the likelihood of withdrawing because of lack of efficacy was the same for olanzapine and placebo. The secondary outcome analyses, which at best would only be useful in generating another study, are confusing because even though time to a return of symptoms (but not diagnosis) was shorter with olanzapine, because of the small numbers the rate of developing new symptoms was not different. Perhaps the most credible finding, although it was not a primary outcome measure either, was that addition of olanzapine was associated with gaining 5–6 kg (11–13 lbs) over the time that patients remained on the medication.

The largest study of an antipsychotic drug in bipolar depression was an industry-sponsored study of olanzapine, which was primarily designed to demonstrate the efficacy of the combination of olanzapine and fluoxetine (Tohen et al., 2003). In this study, 833 patients with bipolar depression (duration 63–82 days) were randomized for 8 weeks to placebo ($N = 377$), olanzapine 5–20 mg ($N = 370$), or various combinations of olanzapine and fluoxetine (doses 6/25, 6/50, or 12/50 mg, respectively; $N = 86$). A major finding was that half the active treatment patients and two thirds of placebo patients dropped out. For the remainder, both active treatments reduced depression scores more than placebo, with effect sizes of 0.32 for olanzapine and 0.68 for the combination of olanzapine and fluoxetine, mostly at higher doses of both medications. The effect size for olanzapine was low enough for this not to be an initial choice for bipolar depression. Given an effect size for fluoxetine plus olanzapine similar to the effect size for fluoxetine alone in unipolar depression, the combination did not appear to increase efficacy of the antidepressant. However, the inference was that the main usefulness of olanzapine was that it prevented fluoxetine-induced mania.

Can this inference be accepted uncritically in a 2-month study? This is a complicated question, about which a clear consensus has yet to emerge. Most bipolar patients who develop mania or hypomania during prospective follow-up are taking antidepressants—and rapid and ultradian cycling begin after a manic or hypomanic episode more frequently than they start out of the blue, but that does not tell us whether antidepressants produced mania/hypomania or rapid cycling, or whether antidepressants just are more likely to be administered to patients who are deteriorating (Altshuler et al., 1995). If a patient starts an antidepressant and immediately becomes manic, it seems more likely that it was caused by the antidepressant, especially if the mania goes away when the antidepressant is discontinued, but once mania or mood cycling begins for whatever reason, they may not stop when the provoking stimulus is discontinued.

By convention, some experimenters have decided that mania that begins within 2 months of starting an antidepressant in someone without a manic past history was induced by the antidepressant, a fairly stringent criterion. But what about hypomania? What about a recurrence of depressive symptoms or more subtle mood swings? And what if mania develops 3 months after starting the antidepressant? Or 3 years? By the most stringent criterion, Altshuler et al. (1995) determined that about half of cases of mania and rapid cycling in a group of patients with complicated mood disorders were attributable to antidepressants and half were attributable to the natural course of the illness, but many of us have seen patients who did well initially on an antidepressant but then got substantially worse after variable periods of time.

The only way to know for sure how frequently antidepressants cause mania or have other adverse consequences for bipolar patients is to randomly assign a group of patients matched for severity and frequency of recurrences to a mood stabilizer plus an antidepressant or a mood stabilizer plus a placebo, and to follow them for an extended period of time, something that no one has yet had the money or the inclination to do. In the meantime, a post-hoc analysis of data from two 3-week controlled trials of olanzapine in mania found worsening of mania scores in 22% of olanzapine-treated patients and 38% of placebo patients (Baker, Milton, Stauffer, Gelenberg, & Tohen, et al., 2003). Aside from the fact that the study was not designed to examine antidepressant-induced mania and did not even involve depressed patients (and it was much too short to justify the conclusion even if it did) we have already seen that retrospective analysis of data obtained for another purpose cannot be used to prove a new idea. Case reports of mania apparently associated with taking olanzapine (Benazzi, 1999; Borysewicz & Borysewicz, 2000; Fitz-Gerald, Pinkofsky, Brannon, Dandridge, & Calhoun, 1999) do not prove that this drug can cause rather than prevent antidepressant-induced mania as the association could have been coincidental, but the clinician who is practicing scientifically will not accept at face value that the fluoxetine-olanzapine combination in bipolar depression is better than or even equivalent to an antidepressant and mood stabilizer combination.

In Altshuler et al.'s (1995) study, established mood stabilizers did not necessarily prevent antidepressant-induced mood destabilization. In contrast, an industry-sponsored randomized, parallel-group yearlong study comparing valproate, lithium, and placebo in patients who recovered from a manic episode within 3 months of open treatment with valproate found that patients taking valproate and an antidepressant were less likely to discontinue treatment because of depression than were patients taking placebo and an antidepressant (Gyulai et al., 2003). The selection of patients for this maintenance study obviously favored valproate responders because it excluded patients who did not improve with acute open treatment and, like most other research of this kind, it did not consider hypomania or mood cycling.

As we have already seen, we should carefully review most of the research that is presented to us, not just industry-sponsored research. A chart review of 1,078 patients with bipolar disorder in the Stanley Foundation network during a naturalistic study of treatment outcome was so influential that it was reported in the *Wall Street Journal* (Altshuler et al., 2003). Of the total group, 549 received an antidepressant for bipolar depression in addition to ongoing treatment with a mood stabilizer. Only 189 patients continued the antidepressant for at least 6 weeks (reasons for discontinuing the antidepressant were not given), and 84 of these responded. The 84 antidepressant responders were divided into those who took the medication for 6 months or less and those who took the antidepressant for more than 6 months; however, it turned out that the former group ($N = 43$) took the antidepressant for an average of 74 days and the latter ($N = 41$) for 484 days.

The risk of depressive relapse was about four times higher in the group that discontinued the antidepressant in a little over 2 months, while the risk of manic relapse was around 18% in both groups. The authors concluded that early antidepressant discontinuation increases the risk of depressive relapse while continuing antidepressants does not increase the risk of mania.

Another interpretation of the data is that only 15% of patients who begin taking an antidepressant or 44% of those who can stay on an antidepressant for at least 6 weeks respond to the medication; at best, the latter rate is similar to the placebo response rate in major depression. In addition, antidepressants may have been withdrawn in a shorter period of time in the "less than 6 months" group because patients were relapsing, or rapid withdrawal of the antidepressant could have caused rebound depression. A major methodological problem in addition to the open method was the use of a single global rating by the primary clinician (CGI [Clinical Global Impressions]-Bipolar) of whether the patient was euthymic, manic, or depressed. As in other studies, hypomania, rapid cycling, and subsyndromal affective dysregulation were not considered. Equally important, the rate of manic recurrence was substantially lower in the entire group than has been reported in other studies from the Stanley Foundation subjects. The statistical method has also been criticized (Soldani, Ghaemi, Tondo, Akiskal, & Goodwin, 2004). The only definitive conclusion that can be drawn from this study that is consistent with clinical experience is that there is a small group of bipolar depressed patients whose moods remain stable for a year or more on the combination of an antidepressant and a mood stabilizer, but it is not yet possible to distinguish in advance these patients from the majority who do not respond to antidepressants or who get worse at some point while taking them.

WHAT ABOUT HOW THE PATIENT IS ACTUALLY DOING?

An important issue to consider in interpreting all clinical trials is what they are actually measuring. We saw on page 45 that response is defined as a 50% reduction of symptoms in depression and mania studies or a 30% symptom reduction of schizophrenia symptom rating scale scores. Remission is usually defined as a depression or mania scale score of 7 or less, often along with a CGI scale score of much or very much improved. However, psychiatric disorders are only diagnosed in *DSM-IV* if symptoms cause distress or interfere with functioning, a dimension that is not considered at all in most studies. While a random sample of the population will probably find a number of people with symptoms such as irritability, insomnia, or difficulty concentrating who are not really ill, patients with a few symptoms who still are not functioning as well as they could, do not do well in relationships, or are persistently withdrawn or dissatisfied, cannot be said to be entirely well.

Many patients—and their therapists—are willing to accept feeling significantly better compared to how they felt before they began treatment, even if they are not totally well. However, this outcome is not really desirable because any residual symptoms, including residual psychosocial dysfunction, increase the risk of major relapse and recurrence. We would therefore like to have treatments that eliminate suffering as completely as possible. Under some circumstances, more than one treatment is needed to achieve this goal, and sometimes treatments should be administered in sequence rather than all at once. However, we do not yet have enough scientific data to tell us what those sequences might be.

The available data provide a good sense of direction in treating uncomplicated disorders such as those more likely to be seen in primary care practice. When treating more complicated disorders, the competent clinician often practices beyond the available controlled data. Rather than providing a license to do whatever the clinician feels might be useful, this truth imposes a profound obligation to remain tied to data from the patient. The scientific practitioner generates a hypothesis about the likely outcome of a particular treatment or combination of treatments and then gathers data as objectively as possible about all important aspects of the patient and the illness. If the clinical hypothesis is not completely confirmed, the clinician must be willing to reassess the situation and change the treatment. The relentless self-examination that is necessary to achieve this goal is difficult to maintain in an era in which we are increasingly taught to trust only the data obtained by others.

6

How to Identify and Deal With Marketing

For years, representatives of every drug company with a product in use in the area brought lunch in rotation once a week for all the residents in our department of psychiatry. At these sessions, the representatives presented their latest material and distributed flashy presentations of recent studies. Having reviewed some of the material presented in this book, the department decided to reorganize relationships with industry. We did not want to prevent all of the representatives' access to the residents, as some departments have done, because we thought that this more extreme approach would not only unnecessarily completely sever ties that can be mutually productive, but it would deprive the residents of the opportunity to learn how to interpret the exchanges that would comprise a significant amount of the continuing education they would be exposed to in practice. Instead, we decided to include interactions with industry representatives in the formal curriculum. In rotation, representatives could make the same presentations (so long as they only handed out peer-reviewed studies), but without the lunch. A faculty member would then discuss the strengths and weaknesses of the presentations in order to illustrate how to interpret the information.

After the first few sessions, the residents were indignant. "This is nothing but marketing," they complained. "What did you think was going on when the same thing happened over pizza?" "That was just lunch. We never paid attention to the presentations." As we have already seen, clinicians' belief—and this includes residents—that they are not influenced by industry marketing, or that even small gifts do not induce a sense of loyalty or obligation to the donor, are not supported by the data.

Apparently, the medium of a simple lunch can obscure the message behind it, or even that a message exists.

MARKETING 101

Drug companies may not be unselfish benefactors of humanity, but they are not malicious conspirators either. They are simply businesses. And like all business, successful companies adhere to basic marketing principles (Hiam, 2004). Understanding a few of these can prepare clinicians to respond to typical marketing maneuvers.

The first rule of marketing is: know your customer. Understanding the customer's needs and ways of thinking makes it possible to develop appealing ways to present the product to the customer. It is important to know how the customer feels and thinks about the product. This helps to plan the best way to convince the customer that the product beats the competition. Depending on the degree to which the customer makes decisions according to logic or feelings, three approaches may be used to sell a product (Hiam, 2004):

1. The informational approach is used when the customer is expected to make a rational decision. This method involves handing out charts and articles, discussing the benefits of the product, and using data to demonstrate its superiority to the competition. It is particularly useful with customers who pride themselves on being well informed and logical.

2. The emotional approach appeals to strong feelings the customer may have about the product line. When Pfizer's atypical antipsychotic, ziprasidone, entered an increasingly lucrative market that had grown to a significant extent due to its predecessors, one of its competitors mounted a campaign against the new kid on the block based on the capacity of ziprasidone to cause prolongation of the QTc (QT interval corrected for heart rate) interval that theoretically could be risky in combination with other drugs that have the same effect and that came on the heels of withdrawal of several antihistamines known to cause more problematic QTc prolongation. The competitor funded talks by experts and took

out ads in psychiatric journals designed to stimulate fears that ziprasidone would have serious cardiac toxicity. The ads were clever in that they did not name ziprasidone, they simply reviewed the dangers of drugs that have this effect without bothering to note that no actual adverse cardiac events had been reported. The campaign was remarkably successful: it not only slowed the entry of ziprasidone into the market, but it kept it off some hospital formularies, maintaining market share for the competitor. The tables were turned when the competitor was found to have the potential to cause diabetes and Pfizer began sponsoring talks about the risks of diabetes with the competitor and clinicians decided that their product was not so bad after all.

3. A combination approach involves both appeals to emotions (e.g., fears of metabolic or cardiac side effects) and information about the benefits of the marketer's product (e.g., data about therapeutic effects and lack of a feared side effect). The decision of how much of each to emphasize will depend on the salesperson's assessment of the customer—in this case, the clinician.

When we are obviously in the role of customer—for example, when buying a car—the salesperson rapidly sizes us up and decides which approach to use. Will we respond better to data presented in charts and articles from automobile magazines about the performance and economy of the product compared to the competition, or will the decision to buy be based on how much we like the way the auto looks and feels or whether it makes us feel safe or prestigious, supplemented by photos and a test drive? Hot dogs and gifts for the kids are used to make us feel good about the dealership. The common practice of splitting the negotiation so that the salesperson carries offers back and forth from a manager helps to maintain the illusion that the salesperson is a friendly ally who only wants the best for us. But that friend has made a highly accurate assessment of how to seal the deal and how much we are willing to pay and has concocted the best sales pitch with the manager.

The sales pitch may be more subtle, but it is just as real in interactions with industry representatives, who use the same standard maneuvers that are part of established marketing principles

(Hiam, 2004). For example, an interesting but inexpensive gift that makes the recipient say "That's cool" or "I can use this" creates a sense of attachment to the product. This is why trinkets such as clocks, umbrellas, and mugs have played such a role in pharmaceutical marketing and why gifts with a special meaning such as a diary with the practitioner's name embossed on it have emotional meaning that gets attached to the company's product. The latest hot gifts being used in a variety of industries that one sees at major professional meetings include mouse pads, flashlights, water bottles, and packaged snacks, all contained in a handy tote bag with a manufacturer's logo on it. The attendee who does not recognize this as a time-tested marketing strategy is like the resident who does not think that pizza could influence prescribing preferences.

Getting someone famous to advertise a product increases its apparent importance. In some cases, public figures actually advertise a product, as when Bob Dole helped to make Viagra a blockbuster drug. A slight modification of this approach is to have a movie star give a lecture at a national meeting on a topic dear to the actor's heart such as bipolar disorder that is related to the product manufactured by the sponsor of the presentation. Just as the manufacturer of a sports car does not have to advertise its product when it sponsors a NASCAR race, it is not necessary to mention the company's product in the talk. In fact, the lecture does not even have to concern psychiatry. Anything that is inspiring or otherwise evokes positive feelings can create a positive association with the manufacturer and its products in the customer's mind.

In the world of medicine, the equivalent of a movie star is a well-known expert. As with the movie star, the expert does not have to actually advertise the product. All that is necessary is to be associated with it in some way, for example, by being in a symposium advertised by a flyer on which the product's or the manufacturer's name appears. Giving the brand a personality also helps. A clever adaptation of the latter principle has been used recently to market eszopiclone. Choosing a name that calls forth images of the moon (Lunesta), advertisements for this medication show a calm butterfly sailing toward its namesake on a peaceful night. The fact that these kinds of maneuvers are more or less obvious does not make them less effective. They are by no means shady or dishonest; they are simply established techniques for selling a product by linking it to a positive image that is evoked along with the image of the product. Recognizing their nature can help us to maintain sufficient distance to interpret whatever information is contained in these presentations.

All products have a life cycle (Hiam, 2004), and pharmaceuticals are no exception. When a new product is introduced, marketing is directed toward telling potential consumers about it and creating a demand for it, often by giving away free samples to entice customers to try it. When the product starts to gain momentum, the product is in its growth phase. During this phase, competitors enter the market and companies marketing similar products jockey for market share. Eventually, the market becomes saturated and simply spreading the good news about the treatment will not create more customers. It is now a priority to hold on to existing customers and steal customers from the competition. Finally, a "death phase" is reached at which something better comes along or, in the case of pharmaceuticals, the patent expires. It may be possible to extend the life span of the product by creating and marketing new uses, which is a motivation for a significant number of Phase IV studies. The decision of whether to extend the patent life by getting approval for new indications or new preparations of the product involves balancing the cost of the necessary FDA studies against the potential additional market. If a new product is not in the pipeline to make up for lost income, the pressure to find a new use for an existing product will be greater.

An interesting example of the extension of the life span of a successful product is the use of a new drug, torcetrapib, which increases levels of HDL cholesterol ("good cholesterol") by inhibiting cholesterol ester transfer protein. Pfizer, the patent holder for the medication, launched a number of studies to determine whether the drug reduces atherosclerotic plaques and reduces the risk of M.I. and stroke (Avorn, 2005). However, the Pfizer trials just compare torcetrapib in combination with another of its drugs, atorvastatin (Lipitor), to atorvastatin alone.

Atorvastatin is currently the best-selling drug in the world (Avorn, 2005). In fact, Lipitor sales account for half of Pfizer's annual profits, and when its patent expires in 2010 this income is likely to decrease as generics become available. If the clinical trials are successful, the FDA will only have data on whether the torcetrapib-atorvastatin is superior to atorvastatin monotherapy. If it is, the FDA will approve torcetrapib only in combination with Lipitor, not in combination with another company's statin or a generic because the approval will be based on a study of a combination tablet, not the two drugs separately. There would be no approval for using torcetrapib with another statin or even with generic atorvastatin when it becomes available. Obviously, clinicians could still combine torcetrapib or a similar drug with any statin based on the data provided by the Pfizer study, but no one but Pfizer could advertise the combination or authorize its representatives to discuss it with physicians. The manufacturer avoids antitrust prohibitions against offering a drug only in combination with another of its products by having the FDA itself do the bundling (Avorn, 2005). Interestingly, publicity about this approach may be leading Pfizer to re-think whether the strategy is worth the bad press.

An approach to anticipating the death phase of a product was demonstrated by Forest Laboratories when it compared its popular antidepressant, citalopram (Celexa), with the new S-enantiomer escitalopram (Lexapro), which it licensed from another company. Because Lexapro has higher affinity for the serotonin transporter, the company claimed that it should be a better antidepressant even though there is no evidence that the degree of affinity for this transporter predicts potency as an antidepressant. As it turned out, the study showed that both drugs were equally effective, but the difference in HDRS scores between Lexapro and placebo was statistically significant earlier in treatment than the difference between Celexa and placebo.

The interpretation of this result was that Lexapro worked faster, but the difference between Celexa and Lexapro in depression rating scale scores was numerically small and of no clinical significance. Nevertheless, the company said that it could not ethically withhold a superior antidepressant and it began conditioning the market to switch products. As soon as Lexapro was approved (not as a superior drug to Celexa or a treatment for refractory depression, but as another SSRI), representatives stopped giving out samples of Celexa and would only provide Lexapro samples. By the time the patent on Celexa ran out, a smooth transition in product loyalty to the manufacturer's new antidepressant had been effected and Lexapro's niche in the antidepressant market was assured.

GUIDELINES FOR INTERACTIONS
WITH INDUSTRY REPRESENTATIVES

If a visit to an auto dealership ends in the customer driving off with a new car, it is obvious that a sale has been made. In the case of a visit by an industry representative to a physician (or anyone else who prescribes medications), the measure of whether the sales pitch worked is whether the physician writes more prescriptions for the representative's product. This measure of marketing effectiveness is easily obtained from local pharmacies. In fact, the representative—and the representative's supervisors—are likely to know more about your prescribing habits than you do. They do not see the names of the patients who receive the prescriptions, but they do know exactly how much of each medication is being prescribed, and by whom. This information is vital in evaluating the effectiveness of the representative in selling the product, and in some circumstances it can determine the representative's future with the company.

The American Medical Association (AMA) recently formally recognized the use by drug companies of the prescribing habits of individual physicians and produced a Web site called the Prescribing Data Restriction Program that provides a place for physicians to ask representatives not to review their prescribing data. At the same time, the AMA says that there may be a "legitimate use of these data by pharmaceutical companies in support of sound health care practices," for example, by providing the samples and educational materials that best suit the physician's prescribing habits and by providing databases that can be used

in research and for "bioterrorism surveillance" (http://www
.amaassn.org/ama/pub/category/12054.html). This kind of fanci-
ful hedge, along with the difficulty physicians experience actually registering for the "do not review" list, may reflect the organization's reluctance to offend the manufacturers who support it
so heavily.

The primary principle of marketing is that companies are in
business to make money by selling their product at a profit. Companies that do not achieve this goal do not survive. And as we
have seen, pharmaceutical companies have not only survived—
they have flourished. If the techniques used by industry representatives were not known to increase sales, they would not use
them. Awareness of this reality and of the specific techniques the
representative uses that are validated by data can prepare the clinician to get the most out of the detailing visit.

In an interesting British report, a general practitioner
recorded and transcribed 10- to 25-minute meetings in his office
with each of eight pharmaceutical representatives (Somerset
et al., 2001). He found that all of these interactions had several
characteristics in common. Each was initiated by the representative, who was deferential to the physician but who was also in
control of the interview. Most of the time, the same kinds of
questions arose and physicians received gifts, promotional material, and other benefits. In contrast with the traditional physician's
role of a knowledgeable, independent expert, the physician's
role was one of potential purchaser, information seeker, and recipient of gifts. The representative's role was one of a friendly,
knowledgeable, and outwardly submissive educator and provider
of gifts whose goal was to be in control of the interview and influence its outcome and whose function as a vendor was paramount
but unstated.

Interactions with the representative followed six scripted
steps. First, the representative gave the practitioner the impression of being the most important person, providing a gift that
serves as a token of appreciation for the doctor's valuable time,
induces a sense of obligation, and functionally if not explicitly
raises the representative's status to that of an equal. The representative then assessed the physician's knowledge, practice, and

use of the product, encouraging the physician to feel correct, but perhaps with the potential to do better. Next, the representative presented selected published research supporting the clinical and cost benefits of the product and initiated a discussion about research, the purposes of which were to assess the physician's skill at critical appraisal. Often, the representative mentioned an expert who was said to be prescribing the medication frequently in order to judge how much the clinician is likely to be influenced by authoritative opinion. If the practitioner resisted this approach, the representative made more extreme statements that conflicted with the practitioner's expertise in order to exert more pressure on the practitioner's opinion, but without directly challenging the physician's expertise.

Having been the object of flattery, sympathy, gifts, and educational opportunities makes the physician feel that the interview was a success. In contrast, the representative measures success by the degree to which a positive relationship and sense of obligation have been induced that create attachment to the representative and with it attachment to the product that will increase the likelihood of prescribing it. The representative takes advantage of a general tendency for people to want to meet with someone who is impressed by their knowledge, sympathetic about the challenges they face, and gives them gifts. This approach follows the established marketing principle of "reciprocity," which holds that a person who is given a gift of any value feels obligated to repay it. Its effectiveness can be validated by following the physician's actual prescribing habits.

Avoiding this kind of interaction completely may prevent being influenced by marketing, but it also deprives the clinician of the actual data contained in the marketing approach. A few simple principles will help clinicians to get the most out of a visit that seems informal but is actually following a structured and well-validated protocol. First and foremost, no matter how cordial and supportive the representative is, no matter how solicitous and helpful, *the representative is not your friend.* Industry representatives are chosen for their interpersonal skills, including their ability to inspire warm feelings. No matter how nice the representative may be as a person, the visit with a clinician is a job, and a job well done will result in the clinician feeling kindly disposed toward the representative and prescribing more of the representative's product. It is not a betrayal for the representative to make use of marketing maneuvers; it is a professional skill that the clinician should not take any more personally than any other well-executed skill.

Many detailing visits include glossy materials and charts provided by the manufacturer. These materials contain concise statements, often with references that are designed to direct the gaze of the busy reader toward one or two key points that validate the product. It is important to bear in mind that these materials are not refereed publications, but marketing tools. The only check on the content is a review by the company's attorneys to be certain that it adheres to FDA guidelines. Such promotional materials bear the same relationship to a neutral description of the product relative to its competition as handouts in an auto showroom do to detailed reviews in car magazines. The split between marketing and other pharmaceutical company divisions that was supposed to make industry information cleaner now requires clinicians to ask for refereed articles to be sent separately, which may seem like more trouble than just looking at the promotional material.

At the same time, *the representative is not a caterer or paymaster*. Many practices carve out time for an industry presentation over lunch, which of course is provided by the representative. It has been common practice for representatives to take physicians out to dinner and sporting events, but the new PhRMA guidelines prohibit favors that are not associated with some sort of promotional or educational activity. Nevertheless, many professional groups still depend on drug companies to provide materials, facilities, and food for professional events. None of these benefits are free. They are provided because they permit access to groups of clinicians. The company keeps track of who was at the event, and the representative is graded on the number of clinicians contacted who are likely to feel an increased sense of loyalty to the product. The interaction between the representative and the practice group would be more straightforward if the company provided an educational grant for a specific activity. The representative's support would be formally acknowledged, and everyone would be aware that the activity is mutually profitable. However, this can no longer be accomplished by the representative as it requires a request to a different division, with a different budget. The representative's funds are limited to clearly promotional events, which are usually organized around a meal.

Promotional meals represent the most reliable remaining venue for the representative to supply something to clinicians along with information about the product. According to the new guidelines, a presentation by a local or national speaker must be promotional. This means that the lecture can only involve the representative's product, and it can only consider FDA-approved indications. The protocol applies equally to dinners or lunches at a restaurant, hospital rounds, university grand rounds, or any other venue. Although it is permissible to answer spontaneous questions after the lecture, the speaker uses slides and handouts prepared by the company in accordance with approved indications. No matter how prominent the speaker, it is important to recognize that in this setting the speaker at most is presenting a glorified package insert. This is not a goal that most universities would like to facilitate.

A draconian approach to industry-sponsored meals was adopted by the Hospital of the University of Pennsylvania (Fallik, 2006). Stating, "I don't think we're entitled to be fed every day," and pointing out that multiple studies demonstrate that small gifts increase the likelihood of prescribing a company's product despite physicians' feelings that their colleagues are influenced by promotional items but they are not, the chief medical officer announced that no drug company meals or gifts would be permitted, at least during regular working hours. Local representatives thought that it would be desirable not to have to provide meals for physicians, but "we found that the only way we could get in to see the doctor was to bring in pizza." Physicians would be discouraged but not prohibited from attending promotional dinners after hours. This was no small loophole, since during the announcement one of the representatives was e-mailing physicians an invitation to a dinner program.

Some physicians do not mind sitting through a lecture on anything for a dinner and the opportunity to interact with their colleagues, but representatives increasingly are recognizing that this approach has the potential to cause as much ill will as loyalty when it becomes apparent that the audience is attending an advertisement. Injury may be added to insult when hospitals and academic departments refuse to give continuing education credits for lectures that are promotional rather than truly educational, as is required for accreditation of CME. As we have already seen, a well-balanced, truly informative presentation that contains new information and makes participants feel that their time has been rewarded creates more goodwill toward the representative and the company than an advertisement for the same product. However, the representative is constrained by company policy. As in all large organizations, it takes a while for information at the bottom to percolate up to the top, but the only way to change the policy may be for physicians and other consumers of industry data to vote with their feet and avoid promotional meals. Remember another cardinal rule of marketing: Give the customers what they want. If we stay away from promotional presentations and only attend lectures that truly represent the work of the speaker, the current policy is more likely to be changed. If we continue to buy the promotional approach that is now in effect, industry will have no reason to change it.

How should clinicians think of industry representatives if not as friends or meal tickets? Perhaps the most appropriate answer is that the representative, like industry itself, should be a *colleague* who brings specific things to the table and who can be a partner in enterprises of benefit to both. As the profession becomes more resistant to the marketing techniques that have been in place until now, it may be possible to develop new collaborations and to develop appropriate mechanisms for financial and scientific support that still meet the marketing needs of industry. For example, leaders of professional groups might begin discussing with representatives whether written requests to them to provide funding for more balanced information combined with not permitting any promotional talks would help them to convince their managers that the promotional talks make the company seem more rather than less invested in directly manipulating physician opinion. Integrating presentations by representatives with objective discussion by faculty experts into resident curricula and grand rounds may be another way to improve industry–clinician collaborations.

If representatives are potential colleagues, it may make sense to sit down with them to discuss how to work together to achieve mutual goals. The representatives want to generate goodwill toward the company, and there is excellent reason to believe that providing quality education will achieve this goal more efficiently than advertising a product. Physicians need funding for specific activities, and changing industry guidelines could make it possible to fund education and research. But unless we are willing to acknowledge that there is in fact no such thing as a free lunch, we can only establish a collegial relationship if we buy our own meals and pens.

OPINION LEADERS

Industry representatives only comprise one arm of marketing influences on prescribing practices (Carpenter, 2002). Sponsored lectures and meetings at which experts present data and opinions occur at academic as well as private sites, not to mention most professional society meetings. Those who attend the annual APA meeting know that the most popular events are industry-sponsored symposia. A great deal of preparation goes into coordinating these symposia, which are usually very well organized, with the best-known speakers and the best slides. Because they are funded by unrestricted educational grants, they are not directly promotional. However, this does not mean that there is no marketing involved.

The amount of money that goes into industry sponsorship of a symposium at the APA meeting reflects awareness that the goodwill and prestige promoted by a valuable program promotes the company's interests more than the cheaper brochures and dinners provided by local representatives. The large audiences at the symposia also provide international exposure for speakers that can help them to market themselves. The quality of these programs should not distract us from realizing that no successful individual or company devotes major resources to an activity that is not potentially profitable. The presentation itself must be of high quality, and obvious material that promotes a particular product will be caught by APA Scientific Program Committee reviewers and the audience, although relative absence of negative data is more difficult to detect. We might ask ourselves how many times a speaker who says that the company's product is inappropriate or no better than anything else for the condition that is the topic of the symposium, or who presents theories of pathogenesis or treatment response that contradict other industry presentations, will be on the next year's program. Success at putting together a truly excellent program and assembling programs that make the sponsor look good (or do not make it look bad) are not mutually incompatible, but both factors should be considered when interpreting the content of large industry-sponsored events. We would not want to restrict or discontinue such programs; we just have to know what to make of the information that is presented and the context in which we hear it.

Industry representatives identify local "opinion leaders" from names that repeatedly come up when asking practitioners whose opinions they value, and by examining who writes the most prescriptions for newer medications (presumably an indication of wanting to be at the cutting edge of psychopharmacology). Local opinion leaders and national figures regularly are invited to participate in industry consultant groups, a service for which the consultant receives a meaningful fee. When the group consists of just a few invitees—say, around 10 or so—the goal is more likely to be to solicit real advice about new research or marketing directions. When several hundred "consultants" attend a meeting in which one presentation after another is made by people who work for the manufacturer or who have other close relationships with it about new research findings by the company, new products in the pipeline, and other exciting developments, the goal is to market the company and its products to influential clinicians who convey their impressions directly or indirectly to their peers. Feedback is solicited from the participants about each major issue that is covered, but its purpose is to make the participants feel that they are part of the process, not to incorporate their suggestions into meaningful strategic changes.

A related large-scale marketing effort involves inviting a few hundred opinion leaders who are interested in giving promotional talks to a speaker training program. The company provides updates on its newest research and then goes through a set of slides that all speakers will use. The slides usually cover general points about disorders for which the company's product is indicated and then summarize selected research and specific points about the company's product and at least some of its competition. The speakers are given the opportunity to discuss the slides and to recommend changes, but the slides are rarely if ever changed. An appealing component of many of these programs is the opportunity to practice giving a brief talk and having it criticized by an expert in public speaking. A successful meeting produces speakers who are better technically, more knowledgeable about the slide content, and focused on the presentation and away from data that contradict its primary points.

The consultant who is invited to a small meeting without extensive presentations of new findings about a product can anticipate an interesting discussion of opinions that may matter to the company and an opportunity to earn the honorarium. Consultants at a large meeting with a highly structured agenda may enjoy the resort where the meeting occurs, and they may hear an interesting talk or two, but it is not likely that their opinion will matter much. If an opinion leader does attend a consultant meeting, it is a good idea to be aware of the primary purpose of the meeting, to critically assess the information that is presented, and to get the most that one can out of the meeting. The opportunity to have one's lecture style critiqued will be very valuable to those attending speaker training sessions at which this service is offered, and it can be good practice to identify the marketing element of the meeting.

SPECIAL JOURNAL ISSUES
AND SYMPOSIA REPORTS

How can certain journals and periodicals afford to provide free subscriptions to virtually all psychiatrists in the United States? The cost of publication is so high that some of the more prestigious journals are prohibitively expensive for all but a few subscribers and libraries, while other highly regarded journals charge authors part of the publication cost (page charges) in order to keep the price of the journal at a reasonable level. Everyone else relies on advertisements. The more advertisements the journal contains, the less the cost of a subscription. Pharmaceutical companies support free journals in two ways: through large advertisements and by buying subscriptions that they then give to favored practitioners as a means of promoting goodwill. A drug company may also pay the entire cost of a special supplement that contains articles summarizing an industry-sponsored symposium on a topic relevant to the manufacturer's product, usually with at least one article directly addressing the product. These articles usually do not reflect original research and do not undergo the same independent review as do regular journal articles.

Despite this limitation, the contents of an industry-supported journal are not purposely skewed to depict the product in a favorable light. Not infrequently, new data or a novel synthesis of ideas makes its way into an industry-supported supplement. However, representatives of the manufacturer, or symposium leaders paid by the manufacturer, may review the article prior to publication and we do not always know what suggestions they have made. In addition, authors of articles in such supplements that suggest that the company's product is not as effective as claimed may not be likely to have articles published in subsequent industry-supported issues. Do journals that contain negative information about a manufacturer or its product have to worry about losing their financial support? Such influences do not inevitably affect the content of the publication, but they can. So we are obligated to exert the effort necessary to review these articles carefully.

The first step in assessing a symposium article is to see who supported it. If the article concerns a product made by the company that paid for the issue, there is probably too great a chance that it will conform to marketing goals to make it worth going through the steps described earlier and in the next chapter to evaluate a research article or a review. If it is on a neutral topic and you trust the author's reputation, the article is best read as an opinion piece, as it is not likely to have been reviewed carefully for accuracy of data, statistical analyses, and inferences. This approach saves the trouble of a careful critical review and allows the reader to get a general impression of the author's views.

7
How to Deal with the Influence of Other Parties

Certain types of articles and activities influence prescribing practices in very profound ways. These activities may not be directly influenced by industry marketing, but they are often based on data obtained in industry-sponsored studies, and they may market a group of clinical ideas beyond the available data. This chapter reviews some of major initiatives and provides a framework for evaluating them.

PRODUCT COMPARISONS

Marketing strategies, as well as some symposia and treatment guidelines, may contain claims of superiority of one product over those of competitors in the same class, usually based on studies that do not directly compare the products, but instead compare results from studies designed to demonstrate the efficacy of each medication compared to placebo. Drugs in the same class (e.g., atypical antipsychotics, anticonvulsants) may have very different actions and effects (McAlister, Laupacis, Wells, & Sackett, 1999), and it is important to be able to determine whether one product is more appropriate than another for a particular patient. However, people are so genetically and psychologically heterogeneous that it is unlikely that average efficacy in a large population will predict specific efficacy in a given patient with a high level of accuracy.

In a recent study (Lee, Kim, Wu, Wang, & Dionne, 2006), patients who just had a wisdom tooth pulled and who had a certain version of the gene (PTG2) for COX-2 had a significantly greater increase expression (induction) of that gene when they took nonsteroidal anti-inflammatory drugs, and these patients had significantly more reduction of pain with the selective COX-2 inhibitor rofecoxib than the nonselective cyclooxygenase-1 (COX-1), COX-2 inhibitor ibuprofen. In contrast, patients with other versions of PTG2 had less induction of the gene by nonsteroidal anti-inflammatory drugs (NSAIDs), and these patients had a better response to ibuprofen, which acts more on COX-1 than COX-2. Like studies that show that lung cancer patients with more expression of a gene for an EGF receptor are more likely to benefit from a drug that blocks that receptor, this study showed that a genetic analysis that can be used in clinical practice could predict which class of medication is more likely to help different patients with the same problem. In psychiatry, pharmacogenomics so far has been used mainly to predict patterns of metabolism of medications like antidepressants, but more specific studies are likely to emerge in the next few years that demonstrate which genes that influence metabolism, receptors, and other drug targets predict a better response in a given individual to which drugs. More detailed studies of correlations of endophenotypes, such as failure of sensory gating, and better studies of response of specific dimensions of illness, such as high rate of recurrence, ultimately will also help to clarify which patient features respond best to which medications.

Until such data become available and easily applied to everyday practice, we have to contend with global comparisons of medications in large groups of patients that can at best give clues to which medications may be initial choices in our patients. These studies may purport to show that a particular medication has better symptomatic outcomes, or they may claim that a medication improves an important domain such as cognitive function or negative symptoms even if other outcomes are not better. We will also see more "noninferiority" studies in which a new medication (e.g., an atypical antipsychotic drug) is shown to be equivalent to an established reference medication in the same class (e.g., haloperidol). There are several levels of reliability of all of these studies, which industry representatives often describe to us or offer to send to us under separate cover (McAlister et al., 1999).

The most reliable comparison of medications is a head-to-head randomized controlled trial with identical patients and clinically important outcomes in which long-term efficacy data are measured. The medications should have been shown to be superior to placebo in previous trials with similar populations and methods.

Showing that a new medication is therapeutically equivalent to another one requires a much larger sample size than standard RCTs. In addition, the same problems can occur in this kind of comparison that occur in clinical trials of single medications. Most important, the doses of the medications being compared may not be truly equivalent. We have already seen how comparisons of new antipsychotic drugs to haloperidol as the reference antipsychotic use haloperidol doses that cause more negative symptoms and cognitive parkinsonism, while haloperidol doses are not adjusted by serum level. Comparisons of new atypical antipsychotic drugs to clozapine do not measure clozapine levels, even though there is probably a correlation between serum level and clinical response (Wahlbeck, Cheine, Essali, & Adams, 1999) and clozapine is usually underdosed in these studies. It is also important to be sure that randomization and blinding were maintained. As with RCTs of a new medication, sample enrichment can greatly limit the generalizability of the results. Failure to use meaningful outcome measures, especially of functioning, and failure to maintain enough patients to the end of the study should also be reasons to take the results with a large grain of salt.

Most randomized trials in psychiatry rely on symptom rating scales much more than measures that are clearly clinically relevant such as how the patient is actually doing, and they only follow patients for a relatively short period of time. A head-to-head randomized comparison of two medications under the conditions just described but without good ratings of long-term functioning in important roles can be useful if a simple outcome measure such as a symptom rating scale score has been shown in good extended randomized studies to be a valid surrogate measure for clinically important outcomes. If a new medication is being compared to an established medication in the same class, at least one drug should have had efficacy demonstrated in long-term trials with clinically important outcomes, which usually extend beyond having a few less symptoms.

A lower level of certainty applies to comparisons of RCTs of different drugs versus placebo in groups of patients who may or may not be similar with respect to illness and risk factors. Lack of comparability of the samples is a particular problem when different manufacturers have enriched study samples for initial response to their product since different patients may respond better to one of these products than another. For the results of different studies to be compared, they should have employed clinically important outcomes or validated surrogate measures and they should have reported ORs or relative risks that can be meaningfully compared. In addition to the limitations of single randomized controlled trials, the main problem with this method is that methods, definitions of endpoints, outcome measures, and duration of treatment usually differ, limiting the comparability of the studies. The findings are much less likely to be useful if surrogate outcome measures such as a single symptom rating scale are used that have not been clearly shown to predict other clinically important outcomes.

Comparisons of subgroup analyses from RCTs of different drugs versus placebo are not as likely as comparisons of main outcome measures to reveal valid differences between the medications. Such comparisons are frequently plagued by statistical weaknesses associated with multiple comparisons, post hoc data mining, and subgroups that are not sufficiently powered to produce meaningful results because they did not involve the primary outcome measure. There is usually insufficient information to be sure whether the subgroups that are compared are really equivalent in these studies. If a representative offers to provide one of these articles or wants to discuss it, it is probably justified to let the offer go.

Comparisons between nonrandomized observational studies and administrative database searches are commonly used to justify assertions that one medication produces better results than another. These kinds of articles represent the least valid kind of data mining because the coding systems used in administrative databases are not designed for research and especially for comparisons of the efficacy of different medications. The methods cannot reassure us that the patients were comparable or that the measures used are valid, and patient compliance is usually not recorded. The primary use of such studies is to generate hypotheses for prospective studies by researchers, not to prove relative efficacy of treatments, and they are usually not worth the clinician's time to read.

CLINICAL REVIEWS

Two types of literature increasingly affect the selection of medications in individual practice as well as global practice standards. Treatment guidelines, which are discussed in the next section, have become a cornerstone of practice. These guidelines depend on systematic reviews, the best of which are written by prominent investigators in the field. As we have already seen, it is rare to find leaders in the field who do not have ties to industry, and some special journal issues containing major reviews are supported by industry. As much as we respect overviews of the field, we should know how to evaluate them critically, especially when they are given to us by industry representatives. The following questions about a systematic review of scientific evidence will help the reader to be sure that treatment decisions will be based on more than the opinion of a respected expert (Oxman, Cook, & Guyatt, 1994):

- Did the overview address a focused clinical question? If the question addressed is not clearly stated, it is only possible to guess whether it is pertinent to patient care. If a specific question is not clear from the title or abstract, skip the article.
- Were appropriate criteria used to select articles to review? The methods that were used to select studies should be stated clearly, as should decisions about the kinds of patients, treatments, and outcomes to include. It is important to be sure that the criteria used to select the studies correspond to the clinical question that led to the review in the

first place and that the reviewer did not choose articles to support a particular bias. Reviews that were commissioned by a drug company or were written by someone who works for the company are more likely to have a bias toward citing positive studies of newer treatments, especially the company's product.

- Is it unlikely that important, relevant studies were missed? At the very least, the authors should have searched bibliographic databases, references cited in articles that are retrieved from the databases, and personal contacts with experts in the area to identify studies that might have been overlooked as well as unpublished studies. As was discussed on pages 17 and 75, omission of unpublished studies increases the chance of publication bias or preferential publication of studies with positive results.

- Was there an assessment of the validity of selected studies? Peer review does not guarantee that the study is valid, even in prestigious journals. Less rigorous studies overestimate the effectiveness of a therapy and bias the review toward a new product.

- Were assessments of studies reproducible? Having multiple reviewers decreases the chance that a single author's viewpoint led to selection of studies that support a particular viewpoint and rejection of those that did not.

- Were methods similar from study to study? If important factors such as patients, methods, diagnoses, treatments, length of follow-up, and outcome measures vary substantially from study to study, it may make no sense to combine them. Tests of homogeneity can be used to determine whether differences among results of individual studies were due to chance or to differences in subjects or study designs. In the latter case, attempting to combine diverse studies may lead to unreliable conclusions.

- Is there a summary outcome measure such as NNT, effect size, or OR that clearly conveys the practical importance of the results? Reviews that only report p values of differences on a particular rating scale score are not as helpful clinically.

- How precise were the results? This can be estimated from the CI of individual or summary statistics. Remember that when 1 or a number close to it is contained in the CI, the likely efficacy of a treatment is not impressive.
- Can the results be applied to a particular clinical setting? An overview of a large number of studies will include results from a diverse group of patients, and if the results are consistent across studies with different populations, they can be assumed to apply to a wide group of patients. However, an individual patient may not be the same as those in the studies, or if studies of different drugs in a class were combined, one of them might have had a larger effect than the others or it might have been more effective in some patients than in others. Conclusions based on comparing patients in one study taking one drug with patients in another study receiving another treatment should be viewed with great skepticism.
- Were all clinically important outcomes considered? A review of studies that only reported symptomatic outcomes or one that did not summarize important adverse events is of limited use for planning real-life clinical practice.
- Are the benefits worth the harms and costs? Ultimately, clinical decision making rests on balancing potential risks and benefits. A comprehensive review that does not help us to assess this balance may provide an impression of global research in the field, but not enough to drive complex treatment decisions in individual patients.

EXPERTS AND CLINICAL GUIDELINES

A decade ago, the APA began publishing clinical practice guidelines, which now cover most of the Axis I disorders. These guidelines have been supplemented by developments in informatics that have facilitated the development of algorithms to guide clinical decision making. Groups such as the Texas Medication Algorithm Project have published their recommendations widely. This group has found that it is possible to get practitioners to adhere to an algorithm, but not that it improves outcomes.

The International Psychopharmacology Algorithm Project is, as its name implies, an international effort to develop automated algorithms that can be applied in multiple settings that has involved a large number of prominent authorities in the field.

As we have already seen, there are significant limitations to the data on which practice guidelines and their visual representations in algorithms are based. Most of the important studies have been supported by industry and have involved patients who have much less complicated disorders than those encountered in specialty practice. Strategies such as sample enrichment, retrospective data mining, and use of secondary outcome measures to prove rather than generate hypotheses make it even more difficult to apply findings that are reported as average results for larger populations to specific patients who might or might not resemble the patients in the study who did well and not the ones who did not do well. Functioning, overall well-being, and residual symptoms, which greatly increase the risk of a major recurrence, are not considered at all in most studies. There are very few practical clinical trials of combination therapies and of patients with refractory and comorbid conditions that would make us completely confident that a practice guideline will apply to a specific patient.

One approach to these limitations is to combine individual guidelines into "meta guidelines" that are not based on specific studies (Villagra, 2004). Since most studies compare one treatment with another in patients who are not yet receiving therapy and not in patients who have failed two or three consecutive treatments, they can guide initial treatment choices better than the next choice if the first one does not work. The Systematic Treatment Alternatives to Relieve Depression (STAR-D) study is the first formal attempt to examine options after the first choice fails, but it can only consider a few sequential treatment choices. Recognized experts in the field are therefore necessary to interpret the data and fill gaps in research. Given the limitations of the data, developing real-life practice guidelines depends on the ability of the expert to draw on broad personal clinical experience as well as published research.

Guidelines are supposed to be just that—recommendations

for treatments that are based on incomplete data and that have the greatest likelihood of efficacy in patients who resemble the patients in studies that led to the guidelines as extended by the experience of the reviewers. However, once they are promulgated, treatment guidelines take on a life of their own. Insurance companies use them to decide whether treatment is worthy of reimbursement, and other reviewers appeal to them to decide whether a given treatment is acceptable. Advocacy groups no less than professional groups now insist on "evidence-based practice" without a true understanding of the nature of the evidence in the evidence base.

To practitioners, administrators, and insurance reviewers in psychiatry, as in other clinical specialties, the term *evidence based* sounds scientific, while anything that is not evidence based is considered inadequate if not incompetent. To maintain credibility, people have gotten into the habit of applying a treatment for which evidence of efficacy exists in an uncomplicated disorder— for example, an SSRI or cognitive behavior therapy in moderate nonpsychotic, nonbipolar depression—and declaring that using the same treatment for another condition, for example, bipolar depression or chronic schizophrenia, is an evidence-based application. It is particularly ironic that clinics that embrace the "recovery movement," which aims to produce the most complete cure for all patients, seem unaware that cure in most studies is defined as symptom reduction rather than the attainment of wellness and that symptomatic remission is not nearly as common as response with evidence based treatments.

In addition to directing our choice of medications, the adoption of practice guidelines has the potential to influence our view of ourselves and what we do. Evaluating treatment strictly according to whatever algorithm quality assurance or utilization reviewers have chosen makes it appear that all that is necessary to provide quality care is to prescribe the right medication or to say that one is performing the right psychotherapy. As the director of an inpatient service said, "I don't have to *think* about anything anymore" (Donald, 2001, p. 427). This clinician (Donald) pointed out that "the practical treatment of each mental illness can be rationalized and streamlined just as the production of products in industry has been streamlined and made economically efficient. . . . The 'algorithmization' of mental illness . . . has become the management of symptoms in a standardized manner," ignoring other important factors in patient care (2001, pp. 430–432).

Donald feels that "managed care algorithms and utilization review represent more than they claim, for they do not represent an advance in scientific knowledge of the natural world of mental illness so much as they reproduce a new moral ideology and actively encourage a notion of personhood and a psychiatric 'science' more suitable to business and consumer culture" (2001, p. 436). A related concern has been that clinicians and reviewers end up spending more time with algorithms and expert opinions than they do with patients (Feinstein & Horwitz, 1997). Patients seem increasingly to agree that the totality of patient experience is being left out of psychiatric treatment, something that is indeed ironic in a field physicians enter because they like learning about and interacting with people. In its 2006 survey of the "State of Depression in America," the Depression and Bipolar Support Alliance (Alliance) pointed out that "treatments that focus solely on symptom relief do not address other aspects of depression such as social functioning, inability to find meaning in life or the desire to be part of one's community" and that "consumers (and their families) often feel frustrated with treatment programs that they have not had a role in selecting," which "often reinforces any feelings that they do not have the power to control their lives" and reduces adherence to treatment and true recovery (2006, p. 48).

Despite these limitations, treatment guidelines are an important advance in formulating a treatment plan that extends beyond individual clinicians' preconceptions and that should consider choices of patients as much as choices of reviewers. Since the most accomplished experts who are recruited for the development of clinical practice guidelines are also recruited for industry-sponsored research and lectures (see Chapter 1), what criteria beyond name recognition can be used to evaluate the guidelines that have proliferated in recent years and that are having such a profound impact on our practice? The Evidence

Based Medicine Working Group and others recommend that practice guidelines be assessed critically with several questions (Guyatt, Sinclair, Hayward, Cook, & Cook, 1995; Hayward, Wilson, Tunis, Bass, & Guyatt, 1995; Richardson & Detsky, 1995). The clinician does not have to remember all of these questions, but groups deciding whether to adopt a practice guideline should be aware of them and individual practitioners may want to refer to them when an attempt is being made to impose practice guidelines that do not seem to make sense.

- What is the primary objective of the guideline? Some guidelines are designed to help with decision making, some to evaluate physician practices, and some to set limits on physician choices. Some are designed for primary care physicians and some for psychiatrists.
- Why was the expert panel recruited for the project? Was it for their knowledge of basic science, their experience with clinical trials, their clinical experience, or some other dimension of expertise?
- Were all important options and outcomes included in the analysis? Most recommendations are essentially decision trees. All relevant decision strategies and all outcomes that matter to patients should be compared, and the clinical strategies should be described from the patient's perspective in enough detail to determine that they are separate and realistic choices. It is important to include the possible consequences of each option, including economic outcomes. If economic analyses were subjected to sensitivity analysis, it is possible to determine whether recommendations might change if cost assumptions change. One obvious example is that if the first choices all cost more than a group of patients is likely to be able to afford, it may be necessary to reorder priorities.
- Was an explicit, meaningful process used to identify, select, and combine evidence? There should be a focused question, explicit inclusion and exclusion criteria, comprehensive search, and reproducible assessment of the validity of the evidence. The search of the literature should be unbiased

and the validity and quality of the studies should be assessed. Randomized controlled trials may not be available to address a specific guideline, or the controlled trials that are available may have significant limitations. The authors should be candid about why they selected these studies and why the limitations of the studies are acceptable. The information that is synthesized should be transformed into quantitative estimates of probabilities ranging from 0 (impossible) to 1 (certain). Each branch of the algorithm should include the probability of outcome with that branch if it can be computed. For example, if there are two possible outcomes and the best estimate for the rate of one of them is 5%, 0.05 is assigned to that branch and 0.95 to the other branch. It may be necessary to adjust data, for example, transforming 5-year survival data into 3-year estimates in order to compare choices. The analysts should then report which data were used and how data were transformed.

• Was a clear process used to consider the relative value of different outcomes, and are there quantitative measures of the value of different choices (utilities)? For example, the relative importance of reducing psychosis or avoiding diabetes depends to a significant extent on which one a patient cares about most. For a given patient, the most credible ratings of the value of a given outcome come from that person. The values are different when guidelines are used for policy determinations that apply to most patients. In this case ratings should come from a survey of the value of different choices in a large group of patients with the disorder in question, from published studies of quality of life ratings for such patients, or at least from a survey of a large group drawn from the general public. For guidelines developed for any purpose, different panel members may value outcomes differently and their sponsorship and biases will help to assess their treatment preferences. A structured process for arbitrating differing values of each intervention reduces undue influence on preferences by individual panel members, especially the chair. However, it is rare to find information in a guideline report about how disagreements about treatment preferences were resolved. When this information is lacking, it is difficult to know how objective the process of creating the guidelines may have been.

- Does the guideline account for major recent developments? Guidelines may be out of date by the time they are published. The date when the final recommendations were made (rather than the publication date) will help to determine whether they should have been updated by now.

- Are the recommendations practical and clinically important? Does one approach lead to a substantial gain, or is the choice between treatments a toss-up? For any clinical outcome, a threshold can be calculated above which the results favor one strategy and below which they favor a different choice. The guideline should specify the threshold level at which the intervention should be used and when it should be a later choice. The reader should be convinced that the benefits of following the recommendations are worth the possible harms and costs. Anticipated reduction of relative and absolute risk would be helpful. The value of the strategy might be measured as quantity or quality of life, or a combined measure such as quality adjusted life years. For example, if a strategy yielded an average increased life expectancy of 5 years, and all 5 years were lived in a state of health rated by patients to have a utility of 0.8 out of 1, quality adjusted life expectancy would be $5 \times 0.8 = 4$ years. All of these values are averages, so some patients will do better than others. A gain in quality-adjusted life expectancy of 2 months or more is considered clinically significant, whereas a gain of a few days is a toss-up. There is less consensus about how to determine the value of psychiatric interventions, and less consensus about how to compute them, making the choices less authoritative.

- How much support do the recommendations have? Are the expected positive and negative outcomes, costs, and consequences sufficient to motivate a change in practice? Levels of evidence for an intervention are graded as:

○ The highest level of support comes from at least one large properly randomized controlled trial or several smaller RCTs, especially when the results of individual studies are similar and all CIs are on one side of the threshold NNT. In other words, all studies agree that the results support that a small enough number of patients would have to be treated to achieve a meaningful effect.

○ Well-designed controlled trials without randomization or RCTs with heterogeneous results, or when the 95% CI overlaps the threshold NNT, are less reliable but still useful.

○ At the next level of reliability are well-designed cohort or case-control studies from more than one center or group and heterogeneous RCTs in which the 95% CIs are all above the threshold number of patients to treat to achieve a meaningful result. Less useful are heterogeneous RCTs in which some CIs are above and some below the threshold NNT.

○ Multiple case series and dramatic results in uncontrolled studies in which the 95% CIs are all above the threshold NNT are more reliable than observational studies in which some studies report CIs that are below the threshold NNT.

○ Opinions of respected authorities based on clinical experience, descriptive studies, or reports of expert committees have the lowest level of solid scientific grounding, but given the dearth of data about complex patients, an experienced clinician may have essential observations and suggestions.

• Was a sensitivity analysis performed, in which the potential impact of uncertainty in the evidence used in the guidelines was determined? There is always uncertainty in clinical decision making because of mixed evidence in the literature and the heterogeneity of both patients and studies. Sensitivity analysis looks at whether the conclusion generated by the decision analysis is affected by uncertainty about the estimates of the likelihood or value of the outcomes. The less precise the estimates of each decision point, the wider the range that should be included in the sensitivity analysis. Failure to acknowledge the realistic uncertainty of recommendation may reflect unanimity of opinion among the reviewers that does not exist in actual practice.

- Has the guideline been subjected to peer review and testing? Confidence in the guideline is increased by external review, clinicians finding the guidelines useful, and similarity to findings by other panels, assuming that the other panels had different members. The best test of usefulness of a guideline is a study of the effect of its implementation on patient outcomes. Since treatment guidelines are considered the last scientific word on clinical practice, there should be scientific evidence that a particular guideline does in fact improve the outcome of treatment. Studies now exist showing some improvement in outcomes of treatment of depression when guidelines are adhered to, but these have mostly been in primary care practices.

- Are the recommendations applicable to patients in your practice, and do patients place the same value on possible outcomes of a given intervention as patients in the studies that were reviewed? This assessment depends on whether the clinical and personal characteristics of patients in the studies used for the decision analysis are similar to those of patients in the practice, and on how your patients would value the outcomes considered in the algorithm. If the patients were different, the clinical variables should be detailed enough to determine where a particular patient might fit in the algorithm and whether the benefit might be the same. If the clinical characteristics of patients in the analysis are not so different from one's own patients that the results should be discarded, it makes sense to proceed with caution.

It should be apparent that practice guidelines therefore do not relieve the clinician of the responsibility to think critically. If anything, it is necessary to evaluate guidelines carefully and discuss their reasoning with patients. The practitioner of evidence-based medicine should understand the patient's total circumstances, identify gaps in knowledge, frame questions as hypotheses, be able to conduct an efficient literature search, assess the evidence, and be prepared to change the approach if it does not work. There is nothing more discouraging than seeing a patient who continued to take a medication that is of no benefit because the treatment is "evidence based."

Since evidence of effectiveness of a treatment in a large population of patients in very well designed clinical trials does not always predict that it is the best intervention for a particular patient in a particular context, the gold standard for determining effectiveness in any individual patient is the N of 1 clinical trial (Guyatt et al., 2000). In this approach, the patient receives a target treatment at one point and a placebo or alternative at another point in random order, with both patient and clinician blind to treatment allocation. The trial continues until patient and clinician agree which is best. This approach is not useful for short-term trials, therapies that cure, or therapies to prevent rare or unique events. With any other kind of evidence, clinicians are generalizing from results in other people to their patients. This is not necessarily bad, so long as doctor and patient continue to be alert to whether the treatment is achieving the outcome they both have agreed is desirable in this particular case.

ADMINISTRATORS AND INSURANCE REVIEWERS

Psychiatrists frequently find themselves in opposition to an insurance reviewer who has decided that clinical guidelines justify denying a particular course of treatment. The psychiatrist may want to use a dose of an antidepressant that is higher than doses used in registration trials and therefore in the package insert, or a combination of medications that has not been proven to be effective because it has never been studied. Or the psychiatrist may want to provide both psychotherapy and pharmacotherapy, as many of us learned was the most effective care, while the insurance company will only pay for 15-minute "med checks" and insists that a nonmedical therapist provide psychotherapy despite evidence that split treatment is no cheaper and certainly no more effective. Perhaps the riskiest interactions occur when the insurance company denies any more hospital days because the patient is no longer acutely suicidal even though the patient is still severely ill and is very likely to become acutely suicidal again after premature discharge. In many of these interactions, the reviewer invokes treatment guidelines and other material to imply (or even state) that the psychiatrist's treatment is below the standard of care.

All insurance companies have a formal process for appealing denials, and the first step often is to demand physician-to-physician review. However, the physician reviewer either works full-time for the insurance company or is frequently utilized by the company for such reviews. Rejection of the appeal does not mean that the reviewing physician's interpretation is consciously biased toward the insurance company, but the reviewer may be more likely to see things from the company's standpoint after performing multiple reviews for them.

There are further levels of appeal by the physician, but it is the patient who has the most power in the process. If enough patients complain to their employers about their poor insurance coverage, the employer may renegotiate the kind of coverage provided to its employers or find another carrier. Complaints by patients to the National Committee on Quality Assurance are used by employers to decide with whom to contract. Helping patients to understand how much power they really have can be an important component of the therapeutic process.

PATIENTS AND FAMILIES

In addition to the explosion of marketing to the public, patients increasingly look to the Internet for information about the latest treatment. Not infrequently, the material they find represents partial understanding of established data or incomplete discussions of a new study or something else that someone heard about. Family members and friends also feel free to give patients advice about treatments they should or should not receive. Armed with impressions that they feel are hot off the press, patients frequently ask for a specific medication they have just heard about. Such requests are understandably common when the current approach is not working well, but some patients who are not doing badly wonder if the latest and greatest thing they have heard about would be better.

A core tenet of informed consent is that the patient chooses the treatment that seems best after understanding the potential risks and benefits of rational options. Deferring to a patient's preference for a particular medication therefore is often entirely appropriate. When a demand for a certain treatment, however, has been stimulated by marketing or incomplete information and it does not make sense—for example, when a patient who has had a difficult time responding to antidepressants and has finally found one that works well wants to change treatments after seeing an advertisement for something better—informed consent becomes more complex.

Much of the time, there is nothing inherently wrong with acceding to a patient's demand for a particular treatment, but it is the clinician's responsibility to evaluate the choice and to help the patient to understand why the data supporting it may not be as straightforward as might be apparent from advertisements or the opinions of friends and relatives. It takes a good deal of skill and empathy to avoid a power struggle and explain the limitations of information that is presented in a brief sound bite or a few sentences on the Internet. Virtually every evening news show has a 2- or 3-minute exposition of a scientific advance that makes it sound as if science is at the same time miraculous and readily grasped. However, a prolonged discussion of why a new SSRI is not necessarily superior to the one that has already been successful requires more than a brief visit. It is the clinician's job to teach the patient restraint in looking for the immediate rapid solution to complex problems.

ADVOCACY GROUPS

The major advocacy groups have developed close relationships with academic leaders and, as we have seen, with industry. As they have become more informed, they have also understandably become more insistent on evidence-based practice. To the extent that academic advisers are anxious for them to appreciate psychiatry's scientific advances, they may be quicker to present the latest study in an easily digestible manner than to explain that the interpretation of the results may not be obvious.

Pointing out the limitations as well as the advances of research in psychopharmacology may create tension with advocacy groups, but it can limit the kind of idealization of science that leads to intense disappointment when an unrealistic promise is not completely fulfilled. As with patients, it may be better to develop a true partnership with advocacy groups that promotes an understanding of all of the dimensions of current knowledge, as is described in Chapter 9.

HOSPITAL ADMINISTRATORS

As insurance coverage for psychiatric inpatient hospitalization has contracted but hospital costs have not, a single unreimbursed day can have a significant impact on hospital finance. Requiring repeated authorizations for each additional day increases the likelihood that payment will be refused because the attending psychiatrist does not have time to talk to a clerk who is following a company algorithm and then either wait on hold for hours while a company physician is located or wait for a return call that comes after the attending has gone to another location.

Hospital administrators are understandably concerned about denials that result from inadequate documentation of medical necessity. However, it is not uncommon these days for attending psychiatrists to receive calls every day about a patient whose well-documented need for continued care is simply refused by the insurance company, which says that the reason for the denial is in keeping with its published protocol. The psychiatrist is then caught between the perception that the patient needs more inpatient care and the likelihood that this care will not be reimbursed by insurance, or by the patient, who cannot afford it. Hospital administrators then put escalating pressure on the psychiatrist to discharge the patient.

No one would reasonably argue that it makes sense to keep a patient in the hospital any longer than is absolutely necessary, but when it is the psychiatrist's judgment that such care is still necessary, conflict with the administrator can become intense. The first thing to do in this circumstance is to obtain a consultation from a colleague agreed to by the administrator and the attending physician. If the verdict is still that the patient needs to stay in the hospital, the potential liability risk to the attending of early discharge may be as great as the potential professional risk of resisting the pressure to get the patient out of the hospital. Under these circumstances, informed consent involves explaining the situation to the patient and planning jointly how to proceed. The patient may not want to stay in the hospital even though the physician believes it is necessary, and in this case the patient may simply want to change doctors. If patient and physician agree that continued hospitalization is needed, the only way for the patient to be discharged would be for the administrator to do so. Obviously, a hospital administrator cannot write a discharge order, but the feeling in administration may be that the physician should no longer work at the hospital. While such actions are risky for hospitals, it may be better to find another job than compromise one's professional judgment when it has been validated by a respected colleague.

8

How to Adapt Your Practice in Light of New Negative Findings

Shortly after initial reports of the efficacy of gabapentin (Neurontin) in bipolar disorder appeared, it rapidly became a first-line treatment, despite the lack of comparisons to standard treatments or even a randomized controlled trial. Thanks to enthusiasm by speakers and by the manufacturer, Neurontin had become a blockbuster drug for multiple indications. In 2004, the company paid $430 million in fines for marketing the drug beyond the data supporting its efficacy (Angell, 2005). Controlled studies of Neurontin in psychiatry showed that it was not more effective than placebo, but many clinicians continued to use it because popular mythology held that it was a good treatment. Their expectation that it should work altered their perception of whether it was actually working. When it became necessary to add other mood stabilizers, the assumption was that the patient simply required combination therapy.

The propensity to continue a treatment one believes in despite evidence from the patient that it is not as effective as it should be creates a kind of self-fulfilling prophecy in which clinicians look for reasons to think that things are getting better and ignore or rationalize contradictory data. Perhaps scores on a depression rating scale have dropped a few points, or perhaps the patient is sleeping better. If the patient still feels empty or suicidal, perhaps it is unrealistic to expect anything better. If the patient does not improve further, it proves the hypothesis. The only way to prevent this kind of outcome is to be aware that any of us is capable of getting stuck in a feedback loop of our own beliefs and therefore to relentlessly examine the data presented by each patient. A scientific method for approaching the clinical encounter is described in the next chapter.

It would be unusual if continued experience with a medication did not dampen its sheen. The Phase III trials that lead to FDA approval are designed to maximize the chance of a positive result and minimize intolerable side effects by eliminating the kinds of complex patients who are seen in most specialty practices. Since many psychiatric disorders evolve over their course, even if a patient resembled patients in a published study when a medication is started, the illness and its response to treatment may change considerably over time so that later in its course it may no longer respond to the same treatment. It is also useful to bear in mind that most published work does not set remission as an a priori primary outcome measure, and even when it does it refers only to symptomatic remission. When we aim to produce a true syndromal remission in our patients, the results with a single treatment do not always look as rosy.

Drazen said, "It is not a failure of the research system when . . . unexpected toxic effects and poor results occur" (2002, p. 1263). But it would be our failure as clinicians not to be vigilant for the inevitable emergence of new adverse findings as well as new cautions about treatment efficacy. There are a number of reasons why RCTs that establish the effectiveness of a medication, especially if they are sponsored by industry, rarely reveal serious side effects that only become apparent after the drug has been in use for some time (Hunter, 2006; March et al., 2005). Most of these studies are too small to detect adverse effects, especially rare ones. For example, a 200-subject trial cannot identify adverse effects that have a frequency of 1 in 500 to 1 in 10,000. Phase III studies in particular are only a few weeks or at most a couple of months long, but it may take years for side effects to emerge, as occurred when it became apparent that some of the atypical antipsychotic medications increase the risk of metabolic disorders such as diabetes.

Just as excluding patients with complex and comorbid disorders, including medical conditions, in industry-sponsored trials excludes patients who would be less likely to respond to the treatment, it excludes patients who are more likely to be susceptible to adverse effects. Sponsors are careful to record and report all side effects promptly, and all serious adverse effects immediately, but these kinds of problems are not as common in Phase III research studies as they are in the clinic. Even common side effects, though, can be missed in the standard registration study. For example, early studies of the SSRIs suggested a rate of sexual dysfunction of 5%, while more systematic studies reported rates of around 50% (Healy, 1999). Why? Because when patients were simply asked whether they had any side effects, many of them did not even realize that sexual dysfunction was caused by the medication. When they were asked specifically about changes in sexual function, the true incidence of the problem became apparent, and it became widely known when the manufacturers of products that do not have this side effect began marketing the information.

HOW ARE NEW SIDE EFFECTS DISCOVERED?

Premarketing safety data are not sufficient to establish definitively the safety of a new medication (McAlister et al., 1999). In postmarketing studies, there are several levels of evidence for examining the safety of new treatments (Levine et al., 1994; McAlister et al., 1999). As is true for efficacy, the most reliable design is a randomized controlled trial in which groups that are similar in all relevant risk factors are assigned to different treatments with the specific aim of determining which is associated with a particular adverse outcome. However, it is difficult to fund a large enough study to detect less common but severe adverse events. No manufacturer is likely to sponsor a study that might prove its product to have unsuspected significant risks, and for the same reason there are virtually no unbiased prospective studies that compare the risks of specific adverse effects in competing medications.

Cohort studies start at exposure status and assess how many patients develop a particular side effect. These studies can follow large groups of patients and are useful for identifying rare but harmful events when randomization of exposure is not possible. In a cohort study, patients select themselves or are selected by their physicians for exposure to the suspected harmful agent. However, there is no reason to assume that exposed subjects are similar to nonexposed subjects with respect to important determinants of outcome. Consider that important GI bleeding occurs in 1.5 per 1,000 person-years of exposure to NSAIDs. A randomized trial to study this side effect would require 6,000 patient-years exposure and 75,000 patient-years per group for sufficient power to test the hypothesis that NSAIDs cause more bleeding than would be expected in the general population. A cohort study of the risk of GI bleeding with NSAIDs would be confounded by the fact that people who take these medications are older, and age is a risk factor for GI bleeding. Additionally, the illnesses that lead people to take NSAIDs could be the real risk factors for GI bleeding.

Some confounding variables that are unequally distributed between groups can be controlled statistically, but since it is difficult to control for the presence of an illness, the result is usually not as strong as in a randomized trial; but it can be intriguing. A cohort study of the risk of diabetes involved a prospective follow-up of all 18,023 MediCal patients under the age of 65 who started taking atypical antipsychotics after December 1998 (Fuller, Shermock, Secic, & Grogg, 2003). The incidence of new onset diabetes mellitus after starting one of these medications was 3.15% with risperidone, 3.04% with quetiapine, and 4.74% with olanzapine. The risk of developing diabetes was 30% higher with olanzapine than risperidone (OR = 1.30), and the risk was greater at higher doses.

Case control studies start with adverse event status and assesses whether subjects with a particular problem were more likely to be exposed to the substance or event in question. In this method, cases are identified who already have the outcome of interest (e.g., a disease, hospitalization, or a side effect) and controls are chosen who are similar with respect to age, sex, concurrent illness, and other factors but do not have the bad outcome. The relative frequency of exposure to the suspected agent is compared among cases and controls. Case control studies are cheaper than prospective studies, and they do not take a long time or involve an enormous number of patients because they examine the prevalence of specific problems in populations who have already been taking a medication for some period of time with those who have not. An association between diethylstilbestrol (DES) and vaginal carcinoma in female offspring of exposed women was demonstrated by comparing young women with vaginal carcinoma who had and did not have DES exposure in utero, controlling for other risk factors such as intrauterine X-ray exposure. A prospective cohort study would have required 20 years and thousands of subjects. However, studies that draw information from large databases such as those from Medicare or HMOs may be limited by lack of information about the temporal relationship between the drug and the adverse event as well as confounding risk factors such as smoking or comorbid illnesses, some of which may not even be in the medical record.

Case control studies have intensified interest in the association of atypical antipsychotics and diabetes. Even the unstructured approach to assessing side effects in the short, early Phase III studies of the atypicals revealed that patients taking drugs such as clozapine and olanzapine gained nearly 10 lbs in just 10 weeks, which was substantially more than with other treatments. However, early case reports of the development of diabetes shortly after starting one of these medications have required further investigation before it can be said that schizophrenia itself is not to blame, since the incidence of diabetes is higher in that disorder than in the general population and it might have been coincidental that diabetes developed when it did. To control for the impact of having schizophrenia, one case control study involved the records of 3.5 million patients in 400 British general practices, including all schizophrenia patients (Koro et al., 2002). Of the 19,637 patients with schizophrenia within this group who did not already have diabetes before taking an antipsychotic drug, 451 developed diabetes within 3 months of starting one of these medications.

Each of the schizophrenia patients who developed diabetes soon after starting an antipsychotic drug was then matched with six schizophrenia patients who never developed diabetes. Compared with schizophrenia patients who did not take antipsychotic drugs, olanzapine increased the risk of diabetes 5.8 times, risperidone increased the risk of diabetes 2.2 times, and neuroleptics increased the risk of diabetes 1.4 times. Starting olanzapine but not risperidone was significantly more likely than starting neuroleptics to be associated with development of diabetes; since clozapine is usually not prescribed by general practitioners and the newer atypical antipsychotics were not in widespread use, the risk of diabetes with these medications was not addressed. The finding was still limited by lack of control for diet, exercise, and severity of schizophrenia, so scientifically the possibility of an interaction of one of these medications with another health factor increasing the risk of diabetes could not be excluded. However, the prudent clinician would start watching more closely for this complication, as well as for more research on the topic.

Industry-sponsored Phase IV studies can detect rare but important adverse effects if they are large enough. However, these studies are more frequently conducted to establish new indications for an established drug, and the same limitations to measuring side effects that affect Phase III studies often apply. Most of the information we get about side effects comes from case reports and case series. Such information can be very useful in calling attention to unsuspected problems, but what appears to be a medication side effect may actually be a manifestation of some other condition or a random phenomenon. The only way to be sure that the medication is to blame is through larger controlled studies. For example, case reports of teratogenicity with Bendectin (a combination of doxylamine, pyridoxine, and dicyclomine used as an antiemetic in pregnancy) led to its withdrawal from the market, but case control studies showed that it was not teratogenic.

HOW TO READ ARTICLES ABOUT
HARMFUL MEDICATION EFFECTS

With increased awareness of the need to keep abreast of new findings, we find ourselves confronted with an increasing number of articles about bad outcomes. A few basic questions can help us to appreciate how concerned we should be (Levine et al., 1994):

- What was the nature of the comparison group? The schizophrenia case control study in which each patient was matched to six controls provided a strong result, but lack of data on diet and other relevant factors was a limitation. A study that controls for most factors that could have accounted for the bad outcome is most desirable but hardly ever feasible, so we have to make our best guess about the validity of the finding.
- How accurate are measures of exposures and outcomes? Were the patients with whom the patients with the bad outcome were matched equally likely to have been exposed to the same risk factors? Recall of exposure is complicated. Issues that commonly make a patient remember more than actually occurred include patient motivation to find an explanation for feeling worse (recall bias) and more aggressive probing by an interviewer (interviewer bias). Reports of increased risk of melanoma in people working with radioactive materials could be a result of "surveillance bias," or more aggressive searching for melanoma in these individuals by physicians, resulting in earlier or more accurate detection of the disease. Reports of a greater risk of being murdered among people who keep a gun in the home would be unreliable if the controls had fewer opportunities to own a gun.
- Was follow-up long and complete enough? It is important to be sure that patients who were lost to follow-up had similar outcomes to those who were not.
- Does the temporal relationship make sense? For example, reports of increased suicidal ideation associated with antidepressants could simply be a manifestation of depression that has not yet responded to the antidepressant (Teicher, Glod, & Cole, 1990). Even new onset suicidal thinking could have appeared after starting the medication because the antidepressant was initiated as depression was worsening. Since a meta-analysis of controlled studies did not support an apparent association of fluoxetine with increased

suicidality (Beasley et al., 1991), the association seems less secure.

- Is there a dose-response relationship? The likelihood of a causal relationship between a suspected agent and an adverse outcome is strengthened if the risk of the adverse outcome is greater the longer the duration of exposure or the greater the stimulus intensity (e.g., total medication dose). This kind of association is clear for tardive dyskinesia but not as much for other adverse effects in which total exposure does not correlate with risk.
- How strong is the association between exposure and outcome? Different measures of this association are used depending on the method:
  - RR is the incidence of the adverse event in the exposed group divided by the incidence in the unexposed group. A RR > 1 suggests increased risk with exposure and a RR < 1 suggests decreased risk with exposure. RR cannot be used in case-control studies in which the proportion of subjects with the outcome is chosen in advance.
  - The OR is the ratio of the odds of a patient with a bad outcome having been exposed to the medication divided by odds of a control patient without the adverse effect having been exposed. The OR approximates the relative risk in case-control studies when the adverse outcome of interest is rare.
  - Larger RR or OR values are required in studies of weaker design such as cohort and case-control studies.
  - RRs and ORs only indicate whether the adverse event is more common in those who took the medication versus those who did not; they do not tell us how frequently the problem occurs
- How precise is the estimate of risk? CIs are used to assess this point. If an association was found between exposure to the medication and an adverse event, the lower end of the CI indicates the minimal strength of the association.
- Are the results applicable to my patients? This determination depends on whether there are clinically important differences between patients in your practice and patients in

the study. For example, some of the estimates of risks of estrogen based on studies of women beginning in the 1970s may not be applicable to patients currently starting the substantially lower doses of estrogen that are recommended now. As with studies of efficacy, studies suggesting a low rate of a particular adverse effect in patients without comorbidity may not apply to patients with the kinds of comorbidities that are encountered in clinical practice.

- What is the magnitude of the risk? This is calculated with the NNH. For example, the CAST showed that over 10 months of treatment following M.I. in an attempt to suppress potentially fatal arrhythmias, the mortality rate was 3% with placebo and 7.7% with Type Ia antiarrhythmics such as quinidine (Levine et al., 1994). The absolute risk increase was 4.7%, and the NNH was $1/0.047 = 21$. In other words, for every 21 patients treated with these drugs for 10 months, there will be one excess death. This was a substantial increase in risk that led to a change in the standard of care away from prescribing Type Ia antiarrhythmics and toward the beta-blockers, which reduced the mortality rate in the same study. The implication for psychiatry was profound, since the tricyclic antidepressants are Type Ia antiarrhythmics. However, since these medications were not included in the CAST study, it is not clear whether they carry the same risk post-M.I.

- Should I stop the exposure? This decision depends on the sum of
  ○ The strength of the studies that demonstrated harm.
  ○ The magnitude of the risk to patients if the exposure continues.
  ○ The potential adverse consequences of reducing or eliminating exposure to the agent.
  ○ Availability of acceptable alternatives to the agent.

For example, while the strength of an association between aspirin use in children and Reye's syndrome is weak and does not clearly demonstrate a causal relationship, the availability of a safe, well-tolerated alternative (acetaminophen) made it easy to recommend that aspirin be avoided in children. On the other hand, the strength of the association between NSAIDs and upper GI bleeding is strong, but the risk is low and, as we have seen, COX-2 inhibitors as alternatives have potential cardiac risks. As a result NSAIDs such as ibuprofen are still used routinely.

HOW NEW INFORMATION EMERGES AND WHAT TO DO ABOUT IT

If we do not idealize new medications, we will remember that there is no such thing as a medication that always works—or one with no potential for harm. A perusal of any clinical trial or package insert makes it clear that even placebos can have significant side effects. All of clinical medicine, regardless of specialty, involves balancing potential risks and benefits of any treatment. Sometimes the risks are apparent immediately, but frequently a good deal of experience is necessary before adverse effects become apparent that develop slowly over time; and low frequency harms require large numbers of patient exposures to reveal themselves.

People tend to accept these realities more readily in other branches of medicine than they do in psychiatry. No one is surprised or files class action suits when cancer treatments cause bone marrow suppression, cardiac damage, or even increased risk of another cancer, but when a few patients developed serious liver disease while taking the antidepressant nefazodone, the manufacturer withdrew the medication from the market to avoid lawsuits (it is still available as a generic). Nomifensine (Merital), an antidepressant that was shown from a case control study to have a risk of causing autoimmune hemolytic anemia before it was released in the U.S., was withdrawn by the manufacturer when further research confirmed the risk. Yet this medication was so uniquely effective for some patients that they would have willingly accepted the risk, especially when it turned out that nothing else ever worked as well for them. For these patients, the risk of depression may have been greater than the risk of the medication.

There are some psychiatric medications that remain on the market despite widely publicized risks. One clear example is clozapine, which causes reversible bone marrow suppression in 1–2% of patients in addition to a number of other side effects that range from cardiac damage to weight gain and diabetes. As a result, it is reserved for refractory schizophrenia and sometimes severe bipolar disorder and aggressive behavior, and patients are monitored carefully. On the other hand, many clinicians avoid prescribing lithium in routine outpatient care because of its potential to cause weight gain, tremor, polyuria, and other side effects, and the need to check blood levels. Why does the ratio of risk to benefit seem too high? Because proprietary medications such as olanzapine and divalproex are marketed as easier to use and safer, even though they can cause weight gain, diabetes, lipid abnormalities, hair loss, and pancreatitis, and the dose cannot be adjusted as precisely as with lithium because there is no clear correlation between blood level and clinical response.

Perhaps the inevitable adverse actions of medications are minimized in psychiatry when most other specialties are up front about them because psychiatrists do not feel as comfortable managing medical risks. If we have not had extensive experience analyzing the outcomes of clinical studies, we may be more likely to accept marketing that makes it sound as if negative effects are negligible compared to positive actions, and industry may get the idea that we respond best to this approach. If we are concerned that patients may not want to take medications if we tell them about all the risks involved, especially if the patient is suspicious or noncompliant, we may market our treatments to our patients in the same manner that the medications are marketed to us.

These approaches will get us (and our patients) to use medications initially, but when something bad happens the rug seems to be pulled out from under our overvaluation and we feel completely disillusioned. Clinicians often forget how much they expected from the treatment and then how disappointed they were, and they simply move on, but patients may not. Lawsuits are not automatically filed in response to an untoward outcome the patient knew to expect, or even because of an unanticipated side effect. Clinicians and manufacturers end up in court when it is perceived that the risk of the side effect was concealed. More complete appreciation of the potential downsides of a new treatment may complicate a patient's initial treatment adherence and it may dampen a physician's initial enthusiasm, but the fact that these treatments can end up harming some people does not mean that they have lost their value. It just means that they are real treatments.

Who can we rely on to keep us updated about newly identified risks of our treatments? To the extent that we have collegial relationships with industry leaders and with representatives, we would expect them to tell us right away when a potential problem is identified. Using diabetes as an example, the responsible representative would let us know that data were emerging suggesting that the product may alter glucose tolerance. The tone of the discussion would not suggest that this was nothing to worry about; indeed, the representative would urge us *to* worry, at least until more information became available, so that we could catch emerging metabolic problems early and deal with them. We would expect this kind of relationship with any supplier of a product for which we represented repeat business, especially when that supplier is part of the health care team.

It is difficult to find research into the frequency with which this kind of productive interchange occurs, but one gets the impression that it is not always the norm. As individuals, many representatives and MSLs are motivated to maintain an honest and open relationship and to have open discussions about the risk/benefit analysis of their product, but not all marketing departments feel the same way. The marketing office responds to objective measures of the success of its efforts, no matter what others may think of them. Robust sales during a marketing campaign that is obviously inappropriate will more than compensate for any physician anger that gets communicated to representatives.

Making it clear to industry representatives that we have much more confidence in products whose necessary blemishes are out in the open than we do in a one-dimensional approach that minimizes the product's flaws may get us more data. However, so long as we do not change our interaction with a company that is not completely open about weaknesses as well as strengths of its product, there is no reason for the company to present us with the latest negative data. One way to get our point across to a company that limits the negative information that is provided to us would be to refuse to see the representative, or the representative's manager, unless they care to show us data that illuminate problems we may encounter with their product as well as its benefits.

Despite the wisdom of providing immediate updates about new negative findings about their products, it does not seem likely that we can rely on industry to do so. Even if it does, clinicians must still seek other sources of data and interpret the data that do become available. A newsletter such as those mentioned in Chapter 9 can be helpful, but before subscribing to one of these for updates on new negative results, readers should peruse a few issues to be sure that the newsletter provides this kind of information rather than general updates on new positive findings.

WHAT TO TELL THE PATIENT

In addition to understanding the nature of the illness and the need for treatment, informed consent depends on receiving accurate information about risks and benefits of a treatment, alternative therapies that competent clinicians would recommend, and the consequences of both treatment and no treatment. With the exception of some emergencies and some severe chronic illnesses and dementias, the decision whether or not to consent to treatment is not impaired by psychiatric disorders; the patient, who suffers any problems caused by a medication, must be the one to decide whether to take it. Informed consent is a dynamic process that evolves with both the state of the illness and new information that emerges. Thus, informed consent cannot be assumed in a patient who does not understand new negative findings.

There are several barriers to keeping patients well-informed. One problem is that there is often not enough time in the brief interactions that are currently covered by insurance and by public sector funding to go into detail about the limitations of new data, especially when it is necessary to correct misconceptions acquired from family and friends or on the Internet. When a patient simply wants to stop a medication immediately after learning of a negative finding, a discussion of the wisdom of this approach can be extensive. Some clinicians are concerned that patients will stop taking a medication or will refuse it in the first place if they hear about any frightening side effects, especially if they misunderstand the finding, and rates of nonadherence are high to begin with in most chronic psychiatric disorders. However, patients who are surprised by a new finding that they hear about first from someone else are not likely to develop the kind of trust that enhances long-term compliance.

A PRACTICAL EXAMPLE

Valproate, an established treatment for bipolar disorder and some forms of anxiety and agitation, rapidly eclipsed mood stabilizers such as lithium thanks not only to its usefulness but also to aggressive marketing by the manufacturer, whose sponsored symposia, journal articles, and advertisements were everywhere as the drug was being rolled out. And the medication seemed ideal. Because it improved sleep and was more sedating, it produced more rapid improvement of mania than lithium, and it did not require such close laboratory monitoring.

In 1993, a year before the publication of the first large randomized controlled trial of valproate for mania (Bowden, Brugger, & Swann, 1994), a study appeared demonstrating that women with epilepsy who started taking valproate as teenagers had an increased risk of developing multiple ovarian cysts and increased androgen activity (Isojarvi, Laatikainen, Pakarinen, Juntunen, & Myllyla, 1993). There was some discussion of this study, which was conducted because the researchers found that valproate alters the conversion of testosterone to estrogen, resulting in abnormal maturation of follicle cells and metabolic abnormalities, but it was not clear that the same would be true for nonepileptic women who started valproate later in life. When asked about the risk, representatives let clinicians know that a new study of bipolar women did not find a significantly increased risk with valproate of polycystic ovary syndrome, a syndrome of ovarian cysts, androgenization (e.g., increased testosterone levels, male pattern baldness, hirsutism), and menstrual abnormalities (Altshuler et al., 2004). What they did not mention was that 8% of women taking valproate but none taking other mood stabilizers had polycystic ovary syndrome, but the study was too small to demonstrate a statistically significant difference. More recently, a study from the STEP-BD comparing 86 bipolar women taking valproate and 144 bipolar women taking other mood stabilizers found that the risk of polycystic ovary syndrome was 7.5 times higher with valproate, this time a significant result (Joffe, 2006). The implication of the finding is magnified by findings that polycystic ovary syndrome increases the risk of developing obesity and diabetes.

Should clinicians have told patients about the contradictory data about the risk to women taking valproate? What should they do now? The most prudent approach would be to let patients know that there could be a risk of ovarian cysts and endocrine dysfunction so that both patient and doctor could be vigilant for the problem. There is still not enough information to predict who might have this side effect or what its long-term implications might be, and this uncertainty may make it difficult for some patients to decide whether the risk is worth taking; but patients have a right to make the best decision they can given the inevitable limitations of available data. If the insurance company does not consider that the time spent discussing these kinds of complex issues with patients is a necessary component of brief "medication checks," some of the maneuvers described on pages 133–134 may prove useful.

9

How to Remain Vigilant

Clinicians have no trouble learning about recalls or dramatic new findings that are publicized in the news or on the Internet. Indeed, patients may hear about new findings before their doctors. Physicians are regularly mailed more detailed warnings when legal advice or the FDA requires it, but by this time most clinicians are already aware of the problems and many patients have heard about them on the Internet. Relying on manufacturers or the government to let us know about new problems with medications, therefore, is not likely to make us the most informed clinicians.

HEALTHY SKEPTICISM

The best tool we have in remaining aware of new developments is reasonable skepticism toward claims about medications, especially when they are made by someone who is selling something—ideas, themselves, or the medication. Skepticism is not the same as cynicism. It is simply not accepting at face value implications that any medication is always the first choice for anything, or that it does not have a potential to harm that can be as great as its potential to help. When we see a study of a new medication or a report of an adverse effect, we will use the rules in Chapters 2, 3, 5, and 8 to analyze the report critically.

Perhaps the most effective application of healthy skepticism is not to rely on industry representatives for updates on clinical applications of their products. Information prepared by the manufacturer must abide by FDA-approved indications, which as we have seen are generally not derived from the kinds of patients most of us see in our practices. Hearsay about what local opinion leaders are supposed to think about a medication is not reliable, since we are much more likely to be told that "Dr. X really likes this medication for treatment-resistant depression" than "Dr. X thinks the medication is a waste of money." Whenever we are told that an expert we admire has made certain statements about a product, it is a good idea to check with that expert to see if the information is being reported accurately. On the other hand, we can probably be more confident in negative information about a representative's product since there is nothing to be gained except credibility in telling us about such information.

These days, lectures sponsored by the representative are less likely to provide meaningful updates than was true in the past. At one time, the local or national experts who were hired to give these talks were able to prepare their own slides and to discuss whatever topic they and their audience chose. The new PhRMA guidelines, however, require that locally sponsored lectures be promotional in order to avoid suggesting unapproved uses of a product. The result is that the talk must center on the manufacturer's product or products and it must not exceed the package insert. If you ask whether you will hear anything you could not learn directly from the manufacturer or the representative, you will be told that the lecturer may have exciting new information during the question and answer session, but you will have to wait until the formal presentation, which cannot deviate from industry-supplied material, is over. It may or may not be worth waiting for the unstructured portion of the program to interact with the lecturer.

The information provided at a promotional talk may amplify information supplied by the representative, but it is not likely to contradict it. A rebellious speaker might cast an entirely new light on industry-supplied material, but experts who are willing to abide by the limits set by the company may be less inclined to risk not being invited to the next talk. If the meals were as sumptuous as they once were, there might be more of a return on the promotional talks, but otherwise the time would be put to more efficient use reading or discussing recent articles.

KEEPING TRACK OF NEW DATA

If we do not rely on industry or the government to keep us up to date, what are we to do? Even if we subscribe to several journals, we are not likely to have time to read all of the articles carefully and at most we may end up perusing the abstracts without appreciating whether the conclusions are justified by the data. And we will still miss major advances reported in journals we do not follow.

One way of keeping up with the flood of new information is to subscribe to one of the newsletters that summarizes recent articles, such as *Journal Watch, Biological Therapies in Psychiatry,* or the *International Drug Therapy Newsletter*. A few basic questions can help to determine how useful the reviews are likely to be. First, does the newsletter contain advertising? Accepting advertisements is the primary means of controlling the cost of the subscription, but it requires that the publisher take extra steps to ensure that the needs of the advertiser do not influence the choice of articles or the way in which they are reviewed. One way to know whether this is an issue is to see whether any reviews are published that cast advertisers' products in a negative light. The same assessment is worth making when a drug company has purchased subscriptions to distribute to clinicians. Such purchases buy goodwill for the company regardless of the content of the newsletter, but it is a good idea to be sure that the newsletter publisher is not unwittingly presenting material that favors the sponsor.

It is also useful to get an overview of the kinds of reports that are summarized. A newsletter that sticks to controlled studies or perhaps large case series is likely to contain more valid information than a newsletter than includes single case reports, letters to the editor, and other uncontrolled observations, especially if any conclusions are drawn beyond suggesting that formal studies should be conducted of the question that was raised in the report. Finally, look carefully at the reviews and see if they provide a balanced interpretation of the data. A summary that raves about a new treatment that was the subject of a single study is less trustworthy than one that summarizes the strengths and weaknesses of the report.

The most reliable, concise source of information about the current status of psychiatric treatments is the *Cochrane Review*. These reviews are conducted by independent investigators who rigorously assess published studies of important treatments. *Cochrane Reviews* can be accessed by subject through Medline and other electronic sites.

The best way for clinicians to put their heads together to learn how to assess recent research critically is through journal clubs. Some industry representatives are willing to fund a journal club around a dinner if it is preceded by a presentation about their product, and this might be worth considering if the representative does not ask to influence the choice of articles. Ask the representative if it is also possible to fund a moderator who is knowledgeable about the research being discussed. The function of a journal club should be not only to summarize recent influential studies but to critique them and place their clinical usefulness in context. The knowledge that comes out of a well-run journal club is clearly worth the effort.

CONSIDERING THE ROLE OF ACADEMIA

Although private research organizations are competing successfully with academic centers for industry-sponsored research, a substantial amount of this research is still being conducted at academic centers. As we have already seen, the majority of industry-sponsored psychiatry studies are designed to get FDA approval and not to investigate anything novel (March et al., 2005). When we review an industry-sponsored Phase III study in which the principle investigator was an academic leader, it will be important to remember that the investigator either did not design the study or participated in the study design in a manner that was satisfactory to the manufacturer. If a prominent academician publishes an investigator-initiated study sponsored by industry, keep in mind that the study may be original, but the company would not support it if it did not have the potential to meet an important marketing goal. This does not automatically mean that the results are suspect, but they must be subject to a higher level of review.

What about academia's educational mission? Traditionally, residents and students have been socialized into relationships with industry through lunches with promotional presentations, gifts, entertainment, dinner lectures, and travel to national meetings. Industry itself has stopped the more blatant activities, but it continues to provide promotional meals and to provide articles and handouts to individual residents. Any kind of access to residents is important for representatives, not only to develop a positive interaction that will persist through the resident's professional life, but also because the representative's supervisor keeps track of the number of visits the representative is able to make.

Some departments of psychiatry have decided to keep representatives away from residents completely. This approach may keep residents free of industry influence, but it does not teach them how to deal constructively with it. The most probable result will be that when they enter practice they will either keep away from industry completely and not have access to any of the positive aspects of interactions with representatives or, more likely, their interactions with industry will be as frequent as anyone else's, but they will not know how to interpret critically the information they receive. In addition, this approach does nothing to redefine the relationship with industry. Any expectation that the rest of this relationship—including support of education and research—will remain the same without any active restructuring of a true partnership is likely to be disappointed.

Can residents and students be taught how to think about the information that is provided to them by industry? One way to achieve this goal would be to eliminate all drug company–sponsored meals to break the association between being fed food and being fed data. Representatives could be invited to make the same kind of presentation they would make to an individual resident or practitioner to a group of residents with a faculty member present. The faculty member would then critically review the presentation and any promotional material that was distributed. A dialogue with the representative could illustrate how to counter deceptive or incomplete interpretations of research. Special symposia or grand rounds could be devoted to the same kind of discussion. For example, representatives with new products or new findings in depression might each make a brief presentation, followed by a discussion by one or more faculty members of the validity of the information that is presented. It might seem that representatives would not be anxious to expose themselves to this kind of debate, but if this is the only access they have to residents and to the extent that they believe in their data, experience shows that it seems like a reasonable way to develop a new partnership.

Many departments of psychiatry rely on industry to fund national speakers at grand rounds, and these speakers have traditionally been chosen from a speaker's bureau provided by the company. Recently, more departments have been asking for unrestricted educational grants that permit them to choose their own speaker. This approach is much less prone to industry influence over grand rounds lectures, but the separation of marketing by representatives and education by MSLs mandated by the new PhRMA guidelines is taking the representatives with whom departments interact every day out of the loop unless a department wants a promotional lecture. Whatever its original intention, this change threatens to force departments to abide by the speaker's bureau or lose industry funding for educational events. The best way to prevent such an outcome is to refuse to choose between any alternatives offered by the company and insist on an unrestricted grant. A departmental committee should decide who to invite based purely on reputation and knowledge of the speaker. If the speaker turns out to be on the company's list, so much the better; but the funding should come from the department, not directly from the company, so that the speaker is not directly beholden to the sponsor. At the same time, industry support for education should be clearly acknowledged, and a company's support of independent education while sacrificing direct advertising should be praised.

WHERE DO WE GO FROM HERE?

The influence of industry in psychiatric research, education, and teaching has been profound, but it has not been entirely bad. If we disabuse ourselves of the notion that a manufacturer should not use established principles to market its products, we can control for the marketing that is inherent in the process as well as the content of interactions with industry. However, a heightened awareness of the nature of information produced and presented by industry leads to a heightened responsibility to evaluate all of the information we receive more critically, and to teach our students how to do the same.

In redefining our relationship with industry, it will be a challenge to retain its more positive dimensions while restricting the more negative ones. We cannot expect industry to support research that has nothing to do with or contradicts it major marketing initiatives, but academia may be able to use funds obtained from conducting Phase III trials to support its own independent investigations. Industry support of education will remain essential, but academia should insist on unrestricted support and more open discussion of the material that is presented, in return for which industry has the opportunity to participate in a more genuine partnership that builds more goodwill, and ultimately more sales, than simply advertising a product.

DTC advertising is one marketing technique that needs redefinition. It can be a public service to inform the public about common mental disorders and their treatability, but it is impossible to present a balanced view of the pros and cons of a particular treatment in a 30-second sound bite in a manner that does anything more than make the consumer want to try the product. Perhaps we should all consider pressuring regulatory agencies to limit television and print advertising to a discussion of the symptoms of a given condition and the fact that many treatments are available. The name of the company that supported the advertisement and even its product could be included, but anything implying that that particular product is better than anything else should be prohibited in the absence of compelling evidence that this is the case—evidence that really only exists for lithium and clozapine, two generic products.

This is indeed an exciting time for psychiatry, not only in the advance of scientific knowledge but in the advance of knowledge about how to understand it. Armed with information about how to interpret new data of any kind, we can become truly scientific practitioners.

REFERENCES

Abramson, J. (2004). *Overdosed America: The broken promise of American medicine.* New York: HarperCollins.

Alliance. (2006). *The state of depression in America.* Chicago: Depression and Bipolar Support Alliance.

Altshuler, L., Rasgon, N. L., Elman, S., Bitran, J. E., Lablarca, R., & Saad, M. (2004). *Reproductive endocrine function in women treated for bipolar disorder: Reproductive hormone levels.* New York: American Psychiatric Association.

Altshuler, L., Suppes, T., Black, D. W., Nolen, W. A., Keck, P. A., Frye, M. A. et al. (2003). Impact of antidepressant discontinuation after acute bipolar depression remission on rates of depressive relapse at 1-year follow-up. *American Journal of Psychiatry, 160,* 1252–1262.

Altshuler, L. L., Post, R. M., Leverich, G. S., Mikalauskas, K., Rosoff, A., Ackerman, L. et al. (1995). Antidepressant-induced mania and cycle acceleration: A controversy revisited. *American Journal of Psychiatry, 152,* 1130–1138.

Anand, G., & Smith, R. J. (2002, August 8). Trial heat: Biotech analysts strive to peek inside clinical tests of drugs. *The Wall Street Journal,* p. A1.

Angell, M. (2005). *The truth about drug companies: How they deceive us and what to do about it.* New York: Random House.

Anonymous (2005, August 17). When doctors advise investors. *The New York Times,* p. 1.

Avorn, J. (2005). Torcetrapib and atorvastatin—should marketing drive the research agenda? *New England Journal of Medicine, 352,* 2573–2576.

Bagby, R. M., Ryder, A. G., Schuller, D. R., & Marshall, M. B. (2004). The Hamilton depression rating scale: Has the gold standard become a lead weight? *American Journal of Psychiatry, 161,* 2163–2177.

Baker, R., Milton, D., Stauffer, V. L., Gelenberg, A. J., & Tohen, M. (2003). Placebo-controlled trials do not find association of olanzapine with exacerbation of bipolar mania. *Journal of Affect Disorders, 73,* 147–153.

Bauer, M., & Mitchner, L. (2004). What is a "mood stabilizer"? An evidence-based response. *American Journal of Psychiatry, 161,* 3–18.

Beasley, C., Dornseif, B. E., Bosomworth, J. C., Sayler, M. E., Rampey, A. H., Heiligenstein, J. H., et al. (1991). Fluoxetine and suicide: A meta-analysis of controlled trials of treatment for depression. *British Medical Journal, 303,* 685–692.

Benazzi, F. (1999). Olanzapine-induced psychotic mania in bipolar schizo-affective disorder [letter to the editor]. *European Psychiatry 14,* 410–411.

Bhandari, M., Busse, J. W., Jackowski, D., Montori, V. M., Schunemann, H., Sprague, S., et al. (2004). Association between industry funding and statistically significant pro-industry findings in medical and surgical randomized trials. *Canadian Medical Association Journal, 170,* 477–480.

Bodenheimer, T. (2000). Uneasy alliance: Clinical investigators and the pharmaceutical industry. *New England Journal of Medicine, 342,* 1539–1544.

Borysewicz, K., & Borysewicz, W. (2000). A case of mania following olanzapine administration. *Psychiatria Polska 34,* 299–306.

Bowden, C., Calabrese, J. R., Sachs, G., Yatham, L. N., Asghar, S. A., Hompland, M., et al. (2003). A placebo-controlled 18-month trial of lamotrigine and lithium maintenance treatment in recently manic or hypomanic patients with bipolar I disorder. *Archives of General Psychiatry 60,* 392–400.

Bowden, C. L., Brugger, A. M., & Swann, A. C. (1994). Efficacy of divalproex vs lithium in the treatment of mania. *Journal of the American Medical Association, 271,* 918–924.

Brennan, T. A., Rothman, D. J., Blank, L., Blumenthal, D., Chimonas, S. C., Cohen, J. J., et al. (2006). Health industry practices that create conflicts of interest: A policy proposal for academic medical centers. *Journal of the American Medical Association, 295,* 429–433.

Calabrese, J. R., Bowden, C., Sachs, G., Yatham, L. N., Behnke, K., Mehtonen, O. P., et al. (2003). A placebo-controlled 18-month trial of lamotrigine and lithium maintenance treatment in recently depressed patients with bipolar I disorder. *Journal of Clinical Psychiatry, 64,* 1013–1024.

Calabrese, J. R., Bowden, C. L., Sachs, G. S., Ascher, J., Monaghan, E., & Radd, G. D. (1999). A double-blind placebo-controlled study of lamotrigine monotherapy in outpatients with bipolar I depression: Lamictal 602 Study Group. *Journal of Clinical Psychiatry, 60,* 79–88.

Campbell, E. G., Louis, K. S., & Blumenthal, D. (1998). Looking a gift horse in the mouth: Corporate gifts supporting life sciences research. *Journal of the American Medical Association, 279,* 995–999.

Carpenter, W. T. (2002). From clinical trial to prescription. *Archives of General Psychiatry, 59,* 282–285.

Cech, T. R. (2005). Fostering innovation and discovery in biomedical research. *Journal of the American Medical Association, 294,* 1390–1393.

Dans, A. L., Dans, L. F., Guyatt, G., & Richardson, S. (1998). How to decide on the applicability of clinical trials results to your patients. *Journal of the American Medical Association, 279,* 545–549.

Diller, L. (2005). Fallout from the pharma scandals: The loss of doctors' credibility? *Hastings Center Report, 35,* 28–29.

Djulbegovic, B., Lacevic, M., Cantor, A., Fields, K. K., Bennett, C. L., Adams, J. R., et al. (2000). The uncertainty principle and industry-sponsored research. *Lancet, 356,* 635–638.

Donald, A. (2001). The Wal-Marting of American psychiatry: An ethnography of psychiatric practice in the late 20th century. *Culture, Medicine and Psychiatry, 25,* 427–439.

Drazen, J. M. (2002). Institutions, contracts, and academic freedom. *New England Journal of Medicine, 347,* 1362–1363.

Dubovsky, S. L. (1994). Beyond the serotonin reuptake inhibitors: Rationales for the development of new serotonergic agents. *Journal of Clinical Psychiatry, 55* (Suppl. 2), 34–44.

Fallik, D. (2006, May 3). Penn bans gifts from drug reps. Doctors' decisions should not be influenced, an official said. *The Philadelphia Inquirer,* pp. 1–2.

Feinstein, A. R. (1995). Meta-analysis: Statistical alchemy for the 21st century. *Journal of Clinical Epidemiology, 48,* 71–79.

Feinstein, A. R., & Horwitz, R. I. (1997). Problems in the "evidence" of "evidence-based medicine." *American Journal of Medicine, 103,* 529–535.

Fitz-Gerald, M. J., Pinkofsky, H. B., Brannon, G., Dandridge, E., & Calhoun, A. (1999). Olanzapine-induced mania [Letter to the editor]. *American Journal of Psychiatry, 156,* 1114.

Fuller, M. A., Shermock, K. M., Secic, M., & Grogg, A. L. (2003). Comparative study of the development of diabetes mellitus in patients taking risperidone and olanzapine. *Pharmacotherapy, 23,* 1037–1043.

Geddes, J., & Goodwin, G. (2001). Bipolar disorder: Clinical uncertainty, evidence-based medicine and large-scale randomised trials. *British Journal of Psychiatry, 178,* S191–S194.

Goodwin, G., Bowden, C., Calabrese, J. R., Grunze, H., Kasper, S., White, R., et al. (2004). A pooled analysis of 2 placebo-controlled 18-month trials of lamotrigine and lithium maintenance in bipolar I disorder. *Journal of Clinical Psychiatry, 65,* 432–441.

Group. (1992). Evidence-based medicine: A new approach to teaching the practice of medicine. *Journal of the American Medical Association, 268,* 2420–2425.

Guyatt, G., Haynes, B., Jaeschke, R., Cook, D. J., Green, L., Naylor, C. D., et al. (2000). EBM: Principles of applying users' guides to patient care. *Journal of the American Medical Association, 284,* 1290–1296.

Guyatt, G. H., Sackett, D. L., & Cook, D. J. (1994). How to use an article about therapy or prevention. *Journal of the American Medical Association, 271,* 59–63.

Guyatt, G., Sinclair, J. C., Hayward, R. S. A., Cook, D. J., & Cook, R. J. (1995). Method for grading health care recommendations. *Journal of the American Medical Association, 274,* 1800–11804.

Gyulai, L., Bowden, C., McElroy, S. L., Calabrese, J. R., Petty, F., Swann, A. C., et al. (2003). Maintenance efficacy of divalproex in the prevention of bipolar depression. *Neuropsychopharmacology, 28,* 1374–1382.

Hammad, T. A., Langhren, T., & Racoosin, J. (2006). Suicidality in pediatric patients treated with antidepressant drugs. *Archives of General Psychiatry, 63,* 332–339.

Hayward, R. S. A., Wilson, M. C., Tunis, S. R., Bass, E. B., & Guyatt, G. (1995). How to use a clinical practice guideline. *Journal of the American Medical Association, 274,* 570–574, 1630–1632.

Healy, D. (1999). The three faces of the antidepressants: A critical commentary on the clinical-economic context of diagnosis. *Journal of Nervous and Mental Disease, 187,* 174–180.

Healy, D. (2006). The latest mania: Selling bipolar disorder. *PLoS Medicine, 3,* e185.

Healy, D., & Cattell, D. (2003). Interface between authorship, industry and science in the domain of therapeutics. *British Journal of Psychiatry, 183,* 22–27.

Healy, D., & Thase, M. E. (2003). Is academic psychiatry for sale? *British Journal of Psychiatry, 182,* 388–390.

Hiam, A. (2004). *Marketing for dummies* (2nd ed.). Indianapolis, IN: Wiley Publishing Inc.

Hollon, M. F. (2004). Direct-to-consumer marketing of prescription drugs: A current perspective for neurologists and psychiatrists. *CNS Drugs, 18,* 69–77.

Horwitz, R. I. (1995). Large-scale randomized evidence: "Large, simple trials and overviews of trials: Discussion. A clinician's perspective on meta-analyses. *Journal of Clinical Epidemiology, 48,* 41–44.

Hunter, D. (2006). First, gather the data. *New England Journal of Medicine, 354,* 329–331.

Isojarvi, J. I., Laatikainen T. J., Pakarinen, A. J., Juntunen, K. T., & Myllyla, V. V. (1993). Polycystic ovaries and hyperandrogenism in women taking valproate for epilepsy. *New England Journal of Medicine, 329,* 1383–1388.

Joffe, H., Cohen, L., Suppes, T., McLaughlin, W. L., Lavori, P., Adams, J. M., et al. (2006). Valproate is associated with new-onset oligoamenorrhea with hyperandrogenism in women with bipolar disorder. *Biological Psychiatry, 59,* 1078–1086.

Jones, P. B., Barnes, T. R. E., Davies, L., Dunn, G., Lloyd, H., Hayhurst, K. P., et al. (2006). Randomized controlled trial of the effect on quality of life of second- vs. first-generation antipsychotic drugs in schizophrenia. *Archives of General Psychiatry, 63,* 1079–1087.

Karpay, K. (2005). Physicians 1, drug-makers 0. *Physicians Practice,* October 2005, p. 10.

Keck, P. E., Jr., McElroy, S. L., Strakowski, S. M., Bourne, B. A., & West, S. A. (1997). Compliance with maintenance treatment in bipolar disorder. *Psychopharmacology Bulletin, 33,* 87–91.

Koro, C. E., Fedder, D. O., L'Italien, G. J., Weiss, S. S., Kreyenbuhl, J., Revick, D. A., Buchanan, R. W. Assessment of independent effect of diabetes among patients with schizophrenia: Population-based case-control study. *British Medical Journal, 325,* 243–245.

Kjaergard, L. L., & Als-Nielsen, B. (2002). Association between competing interests and authors' conclusions: Epidemiological study of randomised clinical trials published in the BMJ. *British Medical Journal, 325,* 249–252.

Kraemer, H. C., & Kupfer, D. J. (2006). Size of treatment effects and their importance to clinical research and practice. *Biological Psychiatry, 59:* 990–996.

Lagomasino, I. T., Dwight-Johnson, M., & Simpson, G. M. (2005). The need for effectiveness trials to inform evidence-based psychiatric practice. *Psychiatric Services, 56,* 649–651.

Lee, Y., Kim, H., Wu, T., Wang, X., & Dionne, R. A. (2006). Genetically mediated interindividual variation in analgesic responses to cyclooxygenase inhibitory drugs. *Clinical Pharmacology & Therapeutics, 79,* 407–418.

Leon, A., Mallinckrodt, C. H., Chuang-Stein, C., Archibald, D. G., Archer, G. E., & Chartier, K. (2006). Attrition in randomized controlled clinical trials: Methodological issues in psychopharmacology. *Biological Psychiatry 59,* 1001–1005.

Levine, M., Walter, S., Lee, H., Haines, T., Holbrook, A., & Moyer, V. (1994). How to use an article about harm. *Journal of the American Medical Association, 271,* 1615–1619.

Lieberman, J. A., Stroup, T. S., McEvoy, J. P., Swartz, M. S., Rosenheck, R. A., Perkins, D. O., et al. (2005). Effectiveness of antipsychotic drugs in patients with chronic schizophrenia. *New England Journal of Medicine, 353,* 1209–1223.

Lynch, T. J., Bell, D. W., Sordella, R., Gurubhagavatula, S., Okimoto, R. A., Brannigan, B. W., et al. (2004). Activating mutations in the epidermal growth factor receptor underlying responsiveness of non-small-cell lung cancer to gefitinib. *New England Journal of Medicine, 350,* 2129–2139.

March, J., Silva, S. G., Compton, M. T., Califf, R., & Krishnan, K. R. R. (2005). The case for practical clinical trials in psychiatry. *American Journal of Psychiatry, 162,* 836–846.

McAlister, F. A., Laupacis, A., Wells, G. A., & Sackett, D. L. (1999). Applying clinical trial results. Part B: Guidelines for determining whether a drug is exerting (more than) a class effect. *Journal of the American Medical Association, 282,* 1371–1377.

McElroy, S. L., Zarate, C. A., Cookson, J., Suppes, T., Haffman, R. F., Ascher, J., et al. (2004). A 52-week, open-label continuation study of lamotrigine in the treatment of bipolar depression. *Journal of Clinical Psychiatry, 65,* 204–210.

Melfi, C. A., Chawla, A. J., Croghan, T. W., Hanna, M. P., Kennedy, S., & Sredl, K. (1998). The effects of adherence to antidepressant treatment guidelines on relapse and recurrence of depression. *Archives of General Psychiatry, 55,* 1128–1132.

Montgomery, J. H., Byerly, M. J., Carmody, T., Miller, D. R., Varghese, F., Holland, R., et al. (2004). An analysis of the effect of funding source in randomized clinical trials of second-generation antipsychotics for the treatment of schizophrenia. *Controlled Clinical Trials, 25,* 598–612.

Moses, H., Dorsey, E. R., Matheson, D. H. M., & Their, S. O. (2005). Financial anatomy of biomedical research. *Journal of the American Medical Association, 294,* 1333–1342.

Motulsky, H. (1995). *Intuitive biostatistics.* New York: Oxford University Press.

Moynihan, R., & Cassels, A. (2005). *Selling sickness: How the world's biggest pharmaceutical companies are turning us all into patients.* New York: Avalon Publishing Group, Inc.

Moynihan, R., Heath, I., & Henry, D. (2002). Selling sickness: The pharmaceutical industry and disease mongering. *British Medical Journal, 324,* 886–890.

Oxman, A. D., Cook, D. J., & Guyatt, G. (1994). How to use an overview. *Journal of the American Medical Association, 272,* 1367–1371.

Perlis, R. H., Perlis, C. S., Wu, Y., Hwang, C., Joseph, M., & Nierenberg, A. A. (2005). Industry sponsorship and financial conflict of interest in the reporting of clinical trials in psychiatry. *American Journal of Psychiatry, 162,* 1957–1960.

Phillips, C. B. (2006). Medicine goes to school: Teachers as sickness brokers for ADHD. *PLoS Medicine, 3,* e182–e184.

Reichardt, T. (2005). Cash interests taint drug advice. *Nature, 437,* 1070–1071.

Richardson, W. S., & Detsky, A. S. (1995). How to use a clinical decision analysis. *Journal of the American Medical Association, 273,* 1610–1613.

Rosenheck, R., Davis, J. M., Evans, D. L., & Herz, A. (2003). Effectiveness and cost of olanzapine and haloperidol in the treatment of schizophrenia: A randomized controlled trial. *Journal of the American Medical Association, 290,* 2693–2702.

Rush, A. J. (2005). Effects of 12 months of vagus nerve stimulation in treatment-resistant depression: A naturalistic study. *Biological Psychiatry, 58,* 355–363.

Schulz, K. F., & Grimes, D. A. (2005). Multiplicity in randomised trials II: Subgroup and interim analyses. *Lancet, 365,* 1657–1661.

Smith, R. (1998). Beyond conflict of interest: Transparency is the key. *British Medical Journal, 317,* 291–292.

Soldani, F., Ghaemi, S. N., Tondo, L., Akiskal, H. S., & Goodwin, F. K. (2004). Relapse after antidepressant discontinuation [Letter to the editor]. *American Journal of Psychiatry, 161,* 1312–1313.

Somerset, M., Weiss, M. K., & Fahey, T. (2001). Dramaturgical study of meetings between general practitioners and representatives of pharmaceutical companies. *British Medical Journal, 323,* 1481–1484.

Steinbrook, R. (2005a). Gag clauses in clinical-trial agreements. *New England Journal of Medicine, 352,* 2160–2162.

Steinbrook, R. (2005b). Wall Street and clinical trials. *New England Journal of Medicine, 353,* 1091–1093.

Teicher, M. H., Glod, C. A., & Cole, J. O. (1990). Emergence of intense suicidal preoccupation during fluoxetine treatment. *American Journal of Psychiatry, 147,* 207–210.

Tiner, R. (2002). The pharmaceutical industry and disease mongering: The industry works to develop drugs, not diseases [Letter to the editor]. *British Medical Journal, 325,* 216.

Tohen, M., Chengappa, K. N., Suppes, T., Baker, R. W., Zarate, C. A., Bowden, C. L., et al. (2004). Relapse prevention in bipolar I disorder: 18-month comparison of olanzapine plus mood stabilizer v. mood stabilizer alone. *British Journal of Psychiatry, 184,* 337–345.

Tohen, M., Vieta, E., Calabrese, J. R., Ketter, T. A., Sachs, G., Bowden, C., et al. (2003). Efficacy of olanzapine and olanzapine-fluoxetine combination in the treatment of bipolar I depression. *Archives of General Psychiatry, 60,* 1079–1088.

Topol, E. J., & Blumenthal, D. (2005). Physicians and the investment industry. *Journal of the American Medical Association, 293,* 2654–2657.

Vainiomaki, M., Helve, O., & Vuorenkoski, L. (2004). A national survey on the effect of pharmaceutical promotion on medical students. *Medical Teacher, 26,* 630–634.

Villagra, V. (2004). Strategies to control costs and quality: A focus on outcomes research for disease management. *Medical Care, 42* (Suppl. 4), III24–30.

Wahlbeck, K., Cheine, M. V., Essali, A., & Adams, C. E. (1999). Evidence of clozapine's effectiveness in schizophrenia: A systematic review and meta-analysis of randomized trials. *American Journal of Psychiatry, 156,* 990–999.

Warner, T., & Roberts, L. W. (2004). Scientific integrity, fidelity and conflicts of interest in research. *Current Opinion in Psychiatry, 2004,* 381–385.

Whiteway, D. E. (2001). Physicians and the pharmaceutical industry: A growing embarrassment and liability. *Wisconsin Medical Journal, 100,* 39–44.

Ziegler, M. G., Lew, P., & Singer, B. C. (1995). The accuracy of drug information from pharmaceutical sales representatives. *Journal of the American Medical Association, 273,* 1296–1298.

Zimmerman, M. E., Chelminski, I., & Posternak, M. A. (2004). Exclusion criteria used in antidepressant efficacy trials: Consistency across studies and representativeness of samples included. *Journal of Nervous and Mental Disease, 192,* 87–94.

INDEX